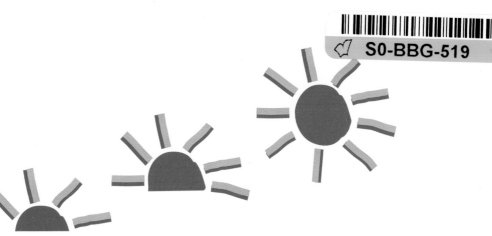

Bright Futures in Practice: Nutrition

Mary Story, Ph.D., R.D.
Katrina Holt, M.P.H., M.S., R.D.
Denise Sofka, M.P.H., R.D.
Editors

Sponsored by
Maternal and Child Health Bureau
Health Resources and Services Administration
U.S. Department of Health and Human Services

Published by
National Center for Education in Maternal and Child Health
Georgetown University

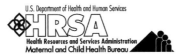

U.S. Department of Health and Human Services
HRSA
Health Resources and Services Administration
Maternal and Child Health Bureau

Cite as

Story M, Holt K, Sofka D, eds. 2000. *Bright Futures in Practice: Nutrition.* Arlington, VA: National Center for Education in Maternal and Child Health.

The mission of the National Center for Education in Maternal and Child Health is to provide national leadership to the maternal and child health community in three key areas—program development, policy analysis and education, and state-of-the-art knowledge—to improve the health and well-being of the nation's children and families. The Center's multidisciplinary staff work with a broad range of public and private agencies and organizations to develop and improve programs in response to current needs in maternal and child health, address critical and emergent public policy issues in maternal and child health, and produce and provide access to a rich variety of policy and programmatic information. Established in 1982 at Georgetown University, NCEMCH is part of the Georgetown Public Policy Institute. NCEMCH is funded primarily by the U.S. Department of Health and Human Services through the Health Resources and Services Administration's Maternal and Child Health Bureau.

Library of Congress Catalog Card Number 00-131028
ISBN 1-57285-063-9

Published by
National Center for Education in Maternal and Child Health
Georgetown University
2000 15th Street, North, Suite 701
Arlington, VA 22201-2617
(703) 524-7802
(703) 524-9335 fax
E-mail: info@ncemch.org
NCEMCH Web site: www.ncemch.org
Bright Futures Web site: www.brightfutures.org

Copies of this publication are available from
National Maternal and Child Health Clearinghouse
2070 Chain Bridge Road, Suite 450
Vienna, VA 22182-2536
(888) 434-4MCH (4624), (703) 356-1964
(703) 821-2098 fax
E-mail: nmchc@circsol.com
NMCHC Web site: www.nmchc.org

This publication has been produced by the National Center for Education in Maternal and Child Health under its cooperative agreement (MCU-119301) with the Maternal and Child Health Bureau, Health Resources and Services Administration, U.S. Department of Health and Human Services.

Table of Contents

Bright Futures Children's Health Charter.. v
What Is Bright Futures? vi
Building Bright Futures... vii
Creating a Lifelong Foundation for Healthy Eating............................ viii
What Is *Bright Futures in Practice: Nutrition*? ix
Bright Futures in Practice: Nutrition Vision and Goals xi
How This Guide Is Organized.. xii
Participants in *Bright Futures in Practice: Nutrition* xiii
Acknowledgments.. xvii
Organizational Support xviii

Introduction 1

Healthy Eating and Physical Activity 3
Nutrition in the Community... 13
Cultural Awareness in Nutrition Counseling 17

Nutrition Supervision Guidelines 21

Infancy 23
Early Childhood... 57
Middle Childhood.. 85
Adolescence... 107

Nutrition Issues and Concerns 133

Breastfeeding... 135
Nutrition and Sports 143
Oral Health.. 152
Vegetarian Eating Practices.. 158
Pediatric Undernutrition... 168
Iron-Deficiency Anemia.. 171
Food Allergy 178
Diabetes Mellitus.. 185
Eating Disorders 190
Obesity 200
Hyperlipidemia 207
Hypertension.. 212
Children and Adolescents with Special Health Care Needs 219

Nutrition Tools 227

Appendix A: Nutrition Questionnaire for Infants................................ 229
Appendix B: Nutrition Questionnaire for Children 232
Appendix C: Nutrition Questionnaire for Adolescents 237
Appendix D: Key Indicators of Nutrition Risk for Children
    and Adolescents... 243
Appendix E: Screening for Elevated Blood Lead Levels...................... 249

Appendix F: Stages of Change—A Model for Nutrition Counseling............... 251
Appendix G: Strategies for Health Professionals to Promote
   Healthy Eating Behaviors 252
Appendix H: Tips for Promoting Food Safety.. 256
Appendix I: Tips for Fostering a Positive Body Image Among
   Children and Adolescents 257
Appendix J: Nutrition Resources.. 258
Appendix K: Federal Food Assistance and Nutrition Programs...................... 266

Bright Futures Children's Health Charter

Throughout this century, principles developed by advocates for children have been the foundation
for initiatives to improve children's lives. Bright Futures participants have adopted these principles in
order to guide their work and meet the unique needs of children and families into the 21st century.

Every child deserves to be born well, to be physically fit, and to achieve
self-responsibility for good health habits.

•

Every child and adolescent deserves ready access
to coordinated and comprehensive preventive, health-promoting, therapeutic,
and rehabilitative medical, mental health, and dental care. Such care is best provided
through a continuing relationship with a primary health professional or team,
and ready access to secondary and tertiary levels of care.

•

Every child and adolescent deserves a nurturing family
and supportive relationships with other significant persons who provide security,
positive role models, warmth, love, and unconditional acceptance.
A child's health begins with the health of his parents.

•

Every child and adolescent deserves to grow and develop
in a physically and psychologically safe home and school environment
free of undue risk of injury, abuse, violence, or exposure to environmental toxins.

•

Every child and adolescent deserves satisfactory housing, good nutrition,
a quality education, an adequate family income, a supportive social network,
and access to community resources.

•

Every child deserves quality child care
when her parents are working outside the home.

•

Every child and adolescent deserves the opportunity to develop ways to cope
with stressful life experiences.

•

Every child and adolescent deserves the opportunity to be prepared for parenthood.

•

Every child and adolescent deserves the opportunity to develop positive values
and become a responsible citizen in his community.

•

Every child and adolescent deserves to experience joy, have high self-esteem,
have friends, acquire a sense of efficacy, and believe that she can succeed in life.
She should help the next generation develop the motivation and habits
necessary for similar achievement.

What Is Bright Futures?

Bright Futures is a vision, a philosophy, a set of expert guidelines, and a practical developmental approach to providing health supervision for children of all ages, from birth through adolescence. Bright Futures is dedicated to the principle that every child deserves to be healthy and that optimal health involves a trusting relationship between the health professional, the child, the family, and the community as partners in health practice.

Bright Futures Mission

The mission of Bright Futures is to promote and improve the health, education, and well-being of infants, children, adolescents, families, and communities.

Bright Futures Project Goals

- Foster partnerships between families, health professionals, and communities
- Promote desired social, developmental, and health outcomes of infants, children, and adolescents
- Increase family knowledge, skills, and participation in health-promoting and prevention activities
- Enhance health professionals' knowledge, skills, and practice of developmentally appropriate health care in the context of family and community

Bright Futures Project Objectives

- Develop materials and practical tools for health professionals, families, and communities
- Disseminate Bright Futures philosophy and materials
- Train health professionals, families, and communities to work in partnership on behalf of children's health
- Develop and maintain public-private partnerships
- Evaluate and refine the efforts

Development of Bright Futures

- Was initiated in 1990 and guided by the Health Resources and Services Administration's Maternal and Child Health Bureau, with additional program support from the Health Care Financing Administration's Medicaid Bureau
- Developed comprehensive health supervision guidelines with the collaboration of four interdisciplinary panels of experts in infant, child, and adolescent health
- Was reviewed by nearly 1,000 practitioners, educators, and child health advocates throughout the United States
- Published *Bright Futures: Guidelines for Health Supervision of Infants, Children, and Adolescents* in 1994
- Launched Building Bright Futures in 1995 to implement the Bright Futures guidelines by publishing practical tools and materials and providing technical assistance and training
- Updated and revised the guidelines for publication in 2000 to incorporate current scientific knowledge in health practice

Funding of Bright Futures

Since its inception in 1990, Bright Futures has been funded by the U.S. Department of Health and Human Services, under the direction of the Maternal and Child Health Bureau.

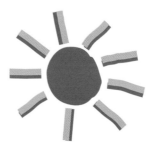

Building Bright Futures

right Futures in Practice: Nutrition is offered in the spirit of health promotion. This comprehensive implementation guide is based on three critical principles consistent with the Bright Futures conceptual framework:

1. Nutrition must be integrated into the lives of infants, children, adolescents, and families.

2. Good nutrition requires balance.

3. An element of joy enhances nutrition, health, and well-being.

The guidelines, philosophy, and goals of the Bright Futures project arose from an understanding that the health of infants, children, and adolescents is affected by their environment and the communities in which they live. In isolation, interventions may have some impact, but in concert with the environment and community, they are more effective and powerful. *Bright Futures in Practice: Nutrition* weaves nutrition principles into all aspects of daily life. It incorporates a clear understanding that food availability, family and cultural customs, and external social pressures (e.g., those created by the media) all influence children's and adolescents' eating behaviors. Integrating good nutrition into the lives of infants, children, and adolescents requires effort in many settings: the home, child care facilities, the school system, and the community. *Bright Futures in Practice: Nutrition* provides suggestions for promoting good nutrition in all of these domains.

Balance is central to good nutrition and good health: the balance of calories, protein, fat, carbohydrates, vitamins, and minerals in the diet; the balance of dependence and independence of the parent and infant, child, or adolescent; the balance of expert advice and common sense; and the balance of cultural norms and secular trends. The contributors to Bright Futures in Practice: Nutrition worked very hard to achieve a balanced presentation about nutrition for infants, children, and adolescents. They have described ways in which food and nutrition can be balanced for good health.

To integrate healthy nutrition and balance into people's lives, a sense of joy is fundamental. The contributors to *Bright Futures in Practice: Nutrition* value the sense of wonder and joy in infants, children, adolescents, families, and communities. Nutrition planning, and preparing and sharing food, are seen as happy events that bring people together—the infant at the mother's breast, the family at the dinner table, and the community at the clam bake.

Bright Futures in Practice: Nutrition provides a thorough overview of nutrition supervision during infancy, early childhood, middle childhood, and adolescence. Each chapter contains current information on nutrition needs as well as techniques for helping children, adolescents, and their families take advantage of this knowledge. We hope that the implementation guide's emphasis on nutritional integration, balance, and joy will improve the lives of infants, children, adolescents, and their families.

Judith S. Palfrey, M.D.
Chair, Building Bright Futures

Creating a Lifelong Foundation
for Healthy Eating

To meet the challenge of developing nutrition guidelines for infants, children, and adolescents, in June 1996, the Bright Futures team convened a multidisciplinary panel of health professionals, including educators, clinicians, public health officials, and representatives from family organizations. The panel focused on two key issues:

1. What do families need to do to promote the nutrition status of infants, children, and adolescents?

2. What do health professionals and communities need to do to become more effective in promoting the nutrition status of infants, children, and adolescents?

The goal was to develop nutrition guidelines for the infancy through adolescence developmental periods. Nutrition guidelines based on the best available scientific research, professional standards, and expert opinions were developed and sent for review to more than 150 individuals from a variety of health agencies and organizations.

Bright Futures in Practice: Nutrition presents the resulting nutrition guidelines and tools designed for use by a wide array of health professionals, including dietitians, nutritionists, nurses, and physicians. The implementation guide can also serve as a practical, educational resource for families and communities.

Bright Futures in Practice: Nutrition emphasizes health promotion, disease prevention, and early recognition of nutrition concerns of infants, children, and adolescents. The guide also highlights how partnerships among health professionals, families, and communities can improve the nutrition status of infants, children, and adolescents.

Bright Futures in Practice: Nutrition builds on the nutrition guidelines presented in *Bright Futures: Guidelines for Health Supervision of Infants, Children, and Adolescents.* The nutrition guide is a practical tool for applying concepts and principles essential to nutrition supervision. It also supports the *Healthy People 2010* objectives for the nation, and can be used to develop and implement programs and policies for the health and well-being of infants, children, and adolescents. *Bright Futures in Practice: Nutrition* represents a vision for the new millennium, a direction for integrating nutrition into health services in the 21st century.

Together, health professionals, families, and communities can work to improve the nutrition status of our nation's infants, children, and adolescents and build a foundation for lifelong healthy eating behaviors—a foundation that encourages infants, children, and adolescents to enjoy eating healthy food and encourages children and adolescents to value family meals and feel good about themselves.

What Is *Bright Futures in Practice: Nutrition?*

Optimal nutrition is important for sustenance, good health, and well-being throughout life. As the relationships among diet, health, and disease prevention have become clearer, nutrition and the promotion of healthy eating behaviors have received increased attention.

The nutrition status of infants, children, and adolescents affects their growth and development and resistance to disease. Lifelong eating behaviors and physical activity patterns are often established in early childhood. Therefore, it is important for children and adolescents to build the foundation for good health by choosing a healthy lifestyle, including practicing healthy eating behaviors and participating in regular physical activity.

A Developmental and Contextual Approach

Nutrition needs to be approached from two perspectives: (1) the development of infants, children, and adolescents and (2) the context of their daily lives and environment. The guidelines in *Bright Futures in Practice: Nutrition* represent a developmental and contextual approach for helping children and adolescents develop positive attitudes toward food and practice healthy eating behaviors.

The developmental approach, which is based on the unique social and psychological characteristics of each developmental period, is critical for understanding children's and adolescents' attitudes toward food and for encouraging healthy eating behaviors.

The contextual approach emphasizes the promotion of positive attitudes toward food and healthy eating behaviors by providing children, adolescents, and their families with consistent nutrition messages. Consistency, combined with flexibility, is essential for handling the challenges of early childhood. During middle childhood and adolescence, it is important for parents to encourage their children and adolescents to become more responsible for their own health and to help them develop the skills they need to practice healthy eating behaviors.

Bright Futures in Practice: Nutrition recommends that food and eating be viewed as both health-enhancing and pleasurable. Food provides more than just energy and sustenance. It holds innumerable symbolic, emotional, social, and personal meanings. Food is connected with nurturing, family, culture, tradition, and celebration. Promoting positive attitudes toward food and healthy eating behaviors in children and adolescents involves recognizing the multiple meanings of food and creating an environment that encourages the enjoyment of food. Family meals are emphasized because they help build on family strengths and promote unity, social bonds, and good communication.

Partnerships Among Health Professionals, Families, and Communities

Encouraging healthy eating behaviors in children and adolescents is a shared responsibility. One of the principles of *Bright Futures in Practice: Nutrition* is that, together, health professionals, families, and communities can make a difference in the nutrition status of infants, children, and adolescents.

Today, many families face the challenges of balancing work and home life and dealing with hectic schedules. Health professionals can help families learn how to fit nutritious meals and snacks into their busy lives. To be most effective, strategies need to be tailored to the family's individual needs.

The family is the predominant influence on children's and adolescents' attitudes toward food and their adoption of healthy eating behaviors. The family exerts this influence by

- Providing the food.

- Transmitting attitudes, preferences, and values about food, which affect lifetime eating behaviors.

- Establishing the social environment in which food is shared.

Parents want to know how they can contribute to their infants', children's, and adolescents' health and are looking for guidance; however, they are faced with contradictory nutrition information. Dietary recommendations can be misunderstood or misinterpreted, especially when adult guidelines are applied to children and adolescents.

Bright Futures in Practice: Nutrition will help health professionals revise standards of practice, promote the development of new nutrition programs, and provide the information children and adolescents need to develop positive attitudes toward food and practice healthy eating behaviors. The guide can serve as a resource for training health professionals and students. Sections of the guide—particularly the Frequently Asked Questions at the end of the Infancy, Early Childhood, Middle Childhood, and Adolescence chapters and the appendices on nutrition risk, food safety, body image, and federal food assistance and nutrition programs—can serve as a resource for educating families.

Throughout the nutrition guide, we use the term "parent" for convenience to refer to the adult or adults responsible for the care of the infant, child, or adolescent. In some situations this person could be an aunt, uncle, grandparent, custodian, or legal guardian.

The community can be invaluable in helping children and adolescents develop positive attitudes about food and practice healthy eating behaviors. *Bright Futures in Practice: Nutrition* can be used in a variety of community settings (e.g., clinics, health and child care centers, hospitals, schools, colleges and universities). Community settings and events that provide a variety of healthy, affordable, and enjoyable foods can be instrumental in communicating positive nutrition messages.

Where We Go from Here

There are many opportunities for promoting the nutrition status of infants, children, and adolescents. It is our sincere hope that *Bright Futures in Practice: Nutrition* will be useful to health professionals, families, and communities as they strive to ensure the health and well-being of the current generation and of generations to come.

Bright Futures in Practice: Nutrition Vision and Goals

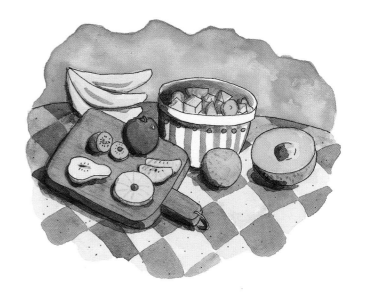

- Improve the nutrition status of infants, children, and adolescents

- Identify desired health and nutrition outcomes that result from positive nutrition status

- Set guidelines to help health professionals promote the nutrition status of infants, children, and adolescents

- Encourage partnerships among health professionals, families, and communities to promote the nutrition status of infants, children, and adolescents

- Describe the roles of health professionals in delivering nutrition services within the community

- Identify opportunities for coordination and collaboration between health professionals and the community

How This Guide Is Organized

Introduction

This section provides information on promoting good nutrition and physical activity as essential components of a healthy lifestyle; establishing a framework for understanding how culture affects food choices and nutrition; and building partnerships among health professionals, families, and communities to promote the nutrition status of infants, children, and adolescents.

Nutrition Supervision Guidelines

This section outlines critical nutrition issues in infancy, early childhood, middle childhood, and adolescence. Each chapter contains an overview of the developmental period; nutrition supervision information tables (including interview questions, screening and assessment, and nutrition counseling); desired health and nutrition outcome; and a list of frequently asked questions with answers that can be used as a handout for families.

Nutrition Issues and Concerns

This section provides an overview of common nutrition issues and concerns that affect infants, children, and adolescents.

Nutrition Tools

This section provides nutrition screening tools, strategies, and resources to help health professionals, families, and communities promote the nutrition status of infants, children, and adolescents.

Participants in *Bright Futures in Practice: Nutrition*

Contributors

Lucy Adams, M.S., C.N.S.
University of California, San Francisco

Irene Alton, M.S., R.D.
Health Start, St. Paul, MN

Paul Casamassimo, D.D.S., M.S.
College of Dentistry, Ohio State
University, Columbus

Catherine Cowell, Ph.D.
School of Public Health, Columbia
University, New York, NY

Peter Dawson, M.D., M.P.H.
School of Medicine, University of
Colorado, Boulder

M. Ann Drum, D.D.S., M.P.H.
Maternal and Child Health Bureau, Health
Resources and Services Administration,
U.S. Department of Health and Human
Services, Rockville, MD

Ardys Dunn, Ph.D., P.N.P., R.N.
School of Nursing, University of
Portland, OR

Larry Gartner, M.D.
Department of Pediatrics, University of
Chicago, IL

Darby Graves, M.P.H., R.D.
WIC Program, Salem, OR

David Heppel, M.D.
Maternal and Child Health Bureau, Health
Resources and Services Administration,
U.S. Department of Health and Human
Services, Rockville, MD

Katrina Holt, M.P.H., M.S., R.D.
National Center for Education in Maternal
and Child Health, Arlington, VA

Janet Horsley, M.P.H., R.D., C.S.
MCH-LEND Program, Virginia Common-
wealth University, Richmond

Daniel Kessler, M.D.
St. Joseph's Hospital and Medical Center,
Phoenix, AZ

Shelley Kirk, M.S., R.D., L.D.
School of Medicine, Children's Hospital
Medical Center, Cincinnati, OH

Emily Loghmani, M.S., R.D., C.D.E.
School of Medicine, Indiana University,
Indianapolis

**Dianne Neumark-Sztainer, Ph.D.,
M.P.H., R.D.**
School of Public Health, University of
Minnesota, Minneapolis

Judith S. Palfrey, M.D.
Children's Hospital of Boston, MA

Peggy Pipes-Johnson, M.P.H., R.D.
Nutrition Consultant, Portland, OR

Denise Sofka, M.P.H., R.D.
Maternal and Child Health Bureau, Health
Resources and Services Administration,
U.S. Department of Health and Human
Services, Rockville, MD

Bonnie Spear, Ph.D., R.D.
Department of Pediatrics, University of
Alabama at Birmingham

Jamie Stang, Ph.D., M.P.H., R.D.
School of Public Health, University of
Minnesota, Minneapolis

Mary Story, Ph.D., R.D.
School of Public Health, University of
Minnesota, Minneapolis

Karen Webber, R.D.N.
Nutrition Consultant, Kelowna, British
Columbia, Canada

Nancy Wooldridge, M.S., R.D.
The Children's Hospital of Alabama,
Birmingham

Executive Steering Committee Members

Eileen Clark
National Center for Education in Maternal
and Child Health, Arlington, VA

Claude Colimon, M.S., R.D.
Health Resources and Services Administration Field Office, Region II, U.S. Department of Health and Human Services, New
York, NY

Catherine Cowell, Ph.D.
School of Public Health, Columbia
University, New York, NY

M. Ann Drum, D.D.S., M.P.H.
Maternal and Child Health Bureau, Health
Resources and Services Administration,
U.S. Department of Health and Human
Services, Rockville, MD

Ardys Dunn, Ph.D., P.N.P., R.N.
School of Nursing, University of
Portland, OR

Katrina Holt, M.P.H., M.S., R.D.
National Center for Education in Maternal
and Child Health, Arlington, VA

Brenda Lisi, M.S., M.P.A., R.D.
Maternal and Child Health Bureau, Health
Resources and Services Administration,
U.S. Department of Health and Human
Services, Rockville, MD
(Formerly of the Food and Nutrition
Service, U.S. Department of Agriculture,
Alexandria, VA)

Pamela Mangu, M.A.
Formerly of the National Center for
Education in Maternal and Child Health,
Arlington, VA

Meri McCoy-Thompson, M.A.L.D.
Formerly of the National Center for
Education in Maternal and Child Health,
Arlington, VA

Judith S. Palfrey, M.D.
Children's Hospital of Boston, MA

Peggy Pipes-Johnson, M.P.H., R.D.
Nutrition Consultant, Portland, OR

Ann Prendergast, M.P.H., R.D.
Maternal and Child Health Bureau, Health
Resources and Services Administration,
U.S. Department of Health and Human
Services, Rockville, MD

Patricia McGill Smith
National Parent Network on Disabilities,
Washington, DC

Denise Sofka, M.P.H., R.D.
Maternal and Child Health Bureau, Health
Resources and Services Administration,
U.S. Department of Health and Human
Services, Rockville, MD

Bonnie Spear, Ph.D., R.D.
Department of Pediatrics, University of
Alabama at Birmingham

Mary Story, Ph.D., R.D.
School of Public Health, University of
Minnesota, Minneapolis

Developmental Panel Members

Lucy Adams, M.S., C.N.S.
University of California, San Francisco

Betsy Anderson
Federation for Children with Special
Needs, Boston, MA

Trina Menden Anglin, M.D., Ph.D.
Maternal and Child Health Bureau, Health
Resources and Services Administration,
U.S. Department of Health and Human
Services, Rockville, MD

Karil Bialostosky, M.S.
National Center for Health Statistics,
Centers for Disease Control and Preven-
tion, U.S. Department of Health and
Human Services, Hyattsville, MD

Linda Sue Black, M.D.
Cobb Pediatrics, Austell, GA

Donna Blum-Kemelor, M.S., R.D.
Food and Nutrition Service, U.S. Department of Agriculture, Alexandria, VA

Joyce Borgmeyer, M.S., R.D.
Health Resources and Services Administra-
tion Field Office, Region XIII, U.S.
Department of Health and Human
Services, Denver, CO

**Mary Sue Brady, D.M.Sc., R.D., C.S.P.,
F.A.D.A.**
School of Medicine, Indiana University,
Indianapolis

Robin Brocato, M.H.S.
Head Start Bureau, Administration on
Children and Families, U.S. Department
of Health and Human Services,
Washington, DC

Susan Brown
Parents as Teachers, Overland, KS

Nan Colvin, R.D.
Piedmont Health District, Farmville, VA

Jane Coury, M.S.N., R.N.
Maternal and Child Health Bureau, Health
Resources and Services Administration,
U.S. Department of Health and Human
Services, Rockville, MD

Kathy Wengen Davis, M.P.H., R.D.
Health Resources and Services Administration Field Office, Region IV, U.S. Department of Health and Human Services,
Atlanta, GA

William Dietz, M.D., Ph.D.
Centers for Disease Control and Preven-
tion, U.S. Department of Health and
Human Services, Atlanta, GA
(Formerly of the New England Medical
Center, Boston, MA)

Shirley Ekvall, Ph.D., R.D., F.A.A.M.D.
Children's Hospital Medical Center,
University of Cincinnati, OH

Valli Ekvall, M.Ed., B.A., R.D., L.D.
Children's Hospital Medical Center,
University of Cincinnati, OH

Arthur Elster, M.D.
American Medical Association,
Chicago, IL

Susan Fay, M.S.N., C.P.N.P., R.N.
Lifelines Children's Hospital,
Clermont, IN

Fannie Fonseca-Becker, M.P.H., R.D.
Nutrition Consultant, Baltimore, MD

Ruth Gitchell, M.S., R.D.
Massachusetts Department of Public
Health, Boston

Jane Goldman, Ph.D.
School of Family Studies, University of
Connecticut, Storrs

Pat Hennessey, M.S., R.D.
WIC Program, Montana Department of
Public Health and Human Services,
Helena

Audrey Janssen, R.D.
Child and Adult Care Food Program,
Bureau of Food and Nutrition Services,
Madison, WI

Marsha Dunn Klein, M.Ed., O.T.R.
Pueblo Pediatric Therapy, Tucson, AZ

William Klish, M.D.
Texas Children's Hospital, Houston

Lloyd Kolbe, M.D.
Centers for Disease Control and Preven-
tion, U.S. Department of Health and
Human Services, Atlanta, GA

Naomi Kulakow, M.A.T.
Center for Food Safety and Applied
Nutrition, Food and Drug Administration,
U.S. Department of Health and Human
Services, Washington, DC

Alan Lake, M.D.
Private Practice Physician, Lutherville, MD

Ruth Lawrence, M.D.
University of Rochester Medical
Center, NY

Brenda Lisi, M.S., M.P.A., R.D.
Maternal and Child Health Bureau, Health Resources and Services Administration, U.S. Department of Health and Human Services, Rockville, MD
(Formerly of the Food and Nutrition Service, U.S. Department of Agriculture, Alexandria, VA)

Helen McClarence, M.Ed., R.D.
Whittier Street Neighborhood Health Center, Roxbury, MA

Peter Miller, M.D., M.P.H.
Maternal and Child Health Consultant, San Anselmo, CA

Marianne Neifert, M.D.
Doctor Mom Presentations, Parker, CO

Dianne Neumark-Sztainer, Ph.D., M.P.H., R.D.
School of Public Health, University of Minnesota, Minneapolis

Susan Nitzke, Ph.D., R.D.
Department of Nutrition Sciences, University of Wisconsin–Madison

Jean Collins Norris, M.S., M.P.H., R.D.
Health Resources and Services Administration Field Office, Region I, U.S. Department of Health and Human Services, Boston, MA

Arthur Nowak, D.M.D.
College of Dentistry, University of Iowa, Iowa City

Donna Oberg, M.P.H., R.D.
Seattle–King County Department of Public Health, Seattle, WA

Annette Peterson, M.S., R.D.
Child and Adult Care Food Program, Montana Department of Public Health and Human Services, Helena

Vivian Pilant, M.S., R.D.
Office of School Food Services, Department of Education, Columbia, SC

Barbara Popper, M.Ed., I.B.C.L.C.
Family Voices, Boston, MA

Mary Ann Raab, M.S.N., C.P.N.P., R.N.
Suburban Pediatrics, Waynesville, OH

Sunita Raynes, M.P.H., R.D.
Maine Ambulatory Care Coalition, Augusta

Jane Mitchell Rees, M.S., R.D.
Department of Pediatrics, University of Washington, Seattle

Karyl Rickard, Ph.D., R.D.
School of Medicine, Indiana University, Indianapolis

Margaret Rodan, M.S.N., M.P.H.
Georgetown University Medical Center, Washington, DC

Lori Rosenblatt, R.D.
WIC Program, Brockton, MA

Charlie Slaughter, M.P.H., R.D.
WIC Program, Department of Human Resources, Portland, OR

Delores Stewart, M.N.S., R.D.
Supplemental Food Program, Mid-Atlantic Region, Robbinsville, NJ

Phyllis Stubbs-Wynn, M.D., M.P.H.
Maternal and Child Health Bureau, Health Resources and Services Administration, U.S. Department of Health and Human Services, Rockville, MD

Carol Suitor, D.Sc., R.D.
Nutrition Consultant, Northfield, VT

Susan Sharaga Swadener, Ph.D., R.D.
Nutrition Consultant, Los Osos, CA

Barbara Turner, B.S., C.D.M.
Broome County Head Start, Binghamton, NY

Frances Vines, M.P.H., R.D.
Health Resources and Services Administration Field Office, Region VI, U.S. Department of Health and Human Services, Dallas, TX

Robin Yeaton Woo, Ph.D., M.B.A.
Center for Food and Nutrition Policy, Georgetown University, Washington, DC

Nancy Wooldridge, M.S., R.D.
The Children's Hospital of Alabama, Birmingham

Organizational Reviewers

Ambulatory Pediatric Association
Sandra Hassink, M.D.

American Academy of Child and Adolescent Psychiatry
David Herzog, M.D.
Alexander Lucas, M.D.

American Academy of Pediatric Dentistry
Steven Adair, D.D.S., M.S.
N. Sue Seale, D.D.S.

American Academy of Pediatrics
Linda Sue Black, M.D.
William Dietz, M.D., Ph.D.
William Klish, M.D.
Alan Lake, M.D.
Ruth Lawrence, M.D.
Peter Miller, M.D., M.P.H.
Marianne Neifert, M.D.
Judith S. Palfrey, M.D.

American College of Nurse-Midwives
Nancy Kuney, R.D., C.N.M.
E. Jean Martin, M.S., M.S.N., C.N.M.

American Dental Association
Carole Palmer, Ed.D., R.D.

American Dental Hygienists' Association
Elizabeth Brutvan, Ed.D., R.D.H.

The American Dietetic Association
Leila Beker, Ph.D., R.D., C.S.P., L.D.
Molly Holland, M.P.H., R.D.
Reed Mangels, Ph.D., R.D., F.A.D.A.
Judith Roepke, Ph.D., R.D.

American Medical Association
Arthur Elster, M.D.
Missy Fleming, Ph.D.

American Nurses Association
Barbara Dunn, Ph.D., C.P.N.P., R.N.

American Public Health Association
Carole Garner, M.P.H., R.D., L.D.
Geraldine Perry, Dr.P.H., R.D.

American School Food Service
Association
Diane Bierbauer, M.S., R.D.
Joanne Kinsey, M.S.
Suzanne Rigby, M.S., R.D.

American School Health Association
Kweethai Neill, Ph.D.
Susan Wooley, Ph.D., C.H.E.S.

Association of Maternal and Child
Health Programs
Kristin Biskeborn, M.P.H., R.D., L.N.
Betsy Emerick, M.S., R.D., L.D.

Association of State and Territorial
Public Health Nutrition Directors
Judy Solberg, M.P.H., M.S., R.D.

Family Voices
Barbara Popper, M.Ed., I.B.C.L.C.

Federation for Children
with Special Needs
Betsy Anderson

March of Dimes
Sarah Smith Carroll, M.P.H.
Richard Johnston, Jr., M.D.

National Association of Pediatric Nurse
Associates and Practitioners
Ardys Dunn, Ph.D., P.N.P., R.N.

National Association of School Nurses
Ann Lowry, B.S., R.N., C.
Joan Thackaberry, M.S.N., R.N., C.S.

National Association of WIC Directors
Beverly Bayan, M.S., R.D.
Stacey Krawczyk, M.S., R.D.

National Parent Network on Disabilities
Patricia McGill Smith

National Parent Teacher Association
Gwen Tucker

Society for Nutrition Education
Won Song, Ph.D., R.D.

Society of Pediatric Nurses
Barbara Keating, M.S., R.N.

U.S. Department of Agriculture, Center
for Nutrition Policy and Promotion
Myrtle Hogbin, B.S., R.D.

U.S. Department of Agriculture, Food
and Nutrition Information Center
Vernice Christian, M.P.H., R.D.

U.S. Department of Agriculture, Food
and Nutrition Service
Donna Blum-Kemelor, M.S., R.D.
Gerry Howell, M.S., R.D.
Avril John, M.S.
Elaine McLaughlin, M.S., R.D.

U.S. Department of Health and Human
Services, National Institutes of Health
Jean Pennington, Ph.D., R.D.

Zero to Three
Peter Dawson, M.D., M.P.H.
Daniel Kessler, M.D.

NCEMCH Project Staff

Carol Adams, M.A.
Director of Publications

Jeanne Anastasi
Senior Editor

Ruth Barzel, M.A.
Senior Editor

Adjoa Burrowes
Senior Graphic Designer

Eileen Clark
Assistant Project Director, Bright Futures

Oliver Green
Senior Graphic Designer

Laura Hjerpe, M.S., M.A.
Reference Librarian

Katrina Holt, M.P.H., M.S., R.D.
Project Director, *Bright Futures in Practice:
Nutrition*

Pamela Mangu, M.A.
Former Project Director, Bright Futures

Anne Mattison, M.A.
Editorial Director

Terry McHugh
Information Specialist

Consultants

Ginny LaFrance
Production Manager

Bonnie Matthews
Illustrator

Meri McCoy-Thompson, M.A.L.D.
Content Editor

Carol Patterson
Production Manager

Beth Rosenfeld
Senior Editorial Consultant

Sharon Schultz
Copyeditor

Gayle Young, M.A.
Copyeditor and Proofreader

Acknowledgments

The Bright Futures project is a major initiative of the Maternal and Child Health Bureau (MCHB), Health Resources and Services Administration, U.S. Department of Health and Human Services. As part of the project's current phase, Building Bright Futures, outstanding leaders in nutrition and health worked together to develop this implementation guide—*Bright Futures in Practice: Nutrition*—a unique and original contribution to the field.

This guide, second in the *Bright Futures in Practice* series, received support and commitment from MCHB, especially from Peter C. van Dyck, associate administrator for maternal and child health; Audrey H. Nora, former MCHB director; Woodie Kessel, former division director; M. Ann Drum, acting division director; David Heppel, division director; and Phyllis Stubbs-Wynn, branch chief.

Judith S. Palfrey, Building Bright Futures chair, also provided leadership and guidance.

Executive Steering Committee members who contributed to this visionary document were Mary Story, Eileen Clark, Claude Colimon, Catherine Cowell, M. Ann Drum, Ardys Dunn, Katrina Holt, Brenda Lisi, Pamela Mangu, Meri McCoy-Thompson, Judith S. Palfrey, Peggy Pipes-Johnson, Ann Prendergast, Patricia McGill Smith, and Bonnie Spear.

This collaborative effort would not have been possible without the leadership, vision, and guidance of Mary Story, chair of *Bright Futures in Practice: Nutrition*. Mary also served as chair of the Adolescent Developmental Panel and prepared and wrote the adolescent section of the guide. It has been an honor to work with her.

Another key person who made this document possible was Katrina Holt, project director, from the National Center for Education in Maternal and Child Health (NCEMCH). Her tireless efforts in organizing the work of the Executive Steering Committee, developmental panels, and reviewers and in writing and editing are very much appreciated.

I would like to acknowledge the contributions of Peggy Pipes-Johnson, chair of the Infancy Developmental Panel; Ardys Dunn; Bonnie Spear, chair of the Middle Childhood Developmental Panel; and Nancy Wooldridge.

These leaders in their fields spent countless hours preparing and writing the developmental sections of the guide.

The following authors also provided outstanding contributions to the guide: Lucy Adams, Irene Alton, Paul Casamassimo, Catherine Cowell, Peter Dawson, Larry Gartner, Darby Graves, Janet Horsley, Daniel Kessler, Shelley Kirk, Emily Loghmani, Dianne Neumark-Sztainer, Jamie Stang, and Karen Webber.

Thoughtful and significant suggestions were contributed by many reviewers, including experts who served on the developmental panels. After reviewers' comments were solicited, a revised draft was sent to representatives from federal agencies and national organizations for review. I would like to acknowledge Ardys Dunn, Brenda Lisi, and Carol Suitor for their efforts in assisting in the review process.

I also extend my deep appreciation to current and former NCEMCH staff members Eileen Clark, Pamela Mangu, and Meri McCoy-Thompson, for their creativity, insight, and perspectives, which can be seen in the strong associations between the foundation document, *Bright Futures: Guidelines for Health Supervision of Infants, Children, and Adolescents*, and this guide. I would also like to recognize the editorial and artistic contributions of NCEMCH Publications Department staff and consultants: Carol Adams, director of publications; Anne Mattison, editorial director; Jeanne Anastasi and Ruth Barzel, senior editors; Beth Rosenfeld, senior editorial consultant; Gayle Young, copyediting and proofreading consultant; Sharon Schultz, copyediting consultant; Adjoa Burrowes and Oliver Green, senior graphic designers; Ginny LaFrance and Carol Patterson, production management consultants; Bonnie Matthews, freelance illustrator; Randy Santos, freelance photographer; and all NCEMCH staff who contributed photographs from personal collections.

It has been a most rewarding experience for me to be a part of this effort.

Denise Sofka, M.P.H., R.D.
Project Officer, *Bright Futures in Practice: Nutrition*
Maternal and Child Health Bureau

Organizational Support

- Ambulatory Pediatric Association
- American Academy of Child and Adolescent Psychiatry
- American Academy of Pediatric Dentistry
- American Academy of Pediatrics
- American Academy of Physician Assistants
- American Alliance for Health, Physical Education, Recreation, and Dance
- American Association for Health Education
- American College of Nurse-Midwives
- American Dental Hygienists' Association
- The American Dietetic Association
- American Medical Association
- American Medical Women's Association
- American Public Health Association
- American School Health Association
- Association of Graduate Programs in Public Health Nutrition
- Association of Maternal and Child Health Programs
- Association of State and Territorial Health Officials
- Association of State and Territorial Public Health Nutrition Directors
- Child Welfare League of America
- CityMatCH
- Family Voices
- Federation for Children with Special Needs
- March of Dimes
- National Association for Sport and Physical Education
- National Association of Community Health Centers
- National Association of County and City Health Officials
- National Association of Pediatric Nurse Associates and Practitioners
- National Association of School Psychologists
- National Association of WIC Directors
- National Organization of Nurse Practitioner Faculties
- National Parent Network on Disabilities
- National Parent Teacher Association
- Society for Adolescent Medicine
- Society for Developmental and Behavioral Pediatrics
- Society for Nutrition Education
- Society of Pediatric Nurses
- Zero to Three

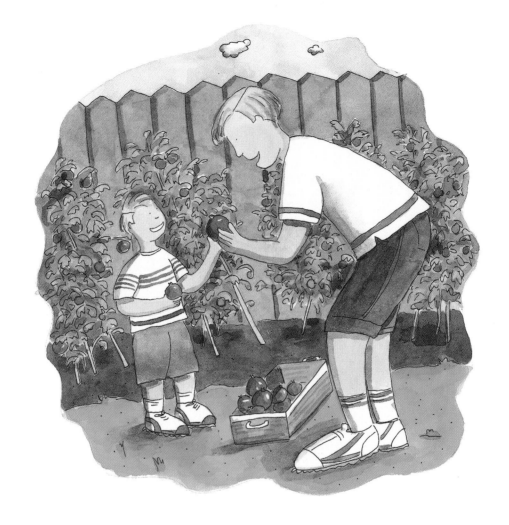

Introduction

HEALTHY EATING AND PHYSICAL ACTIVITY

Healthy eating and physical activity are essential at all stages of life. They are especially important for the growth and development of infants, children, and adolescents. Optimal nutrition and regular physical activity can prevent health problems such as iron-deficiency anemia, obesity, eating disorders, undernutrition, and dental caries. Over the long term, they can help lower the risk of developing chronic disease (e.g., heart disease, certain cancers, diabetes mellitus, stroke, osteoporosis) or risk factors for disease (e.g., obesity, high blood pressure, high blood cholesterol levels).

Unfortunately, there are many barriers to healthy eating. High-fat, high-sugar, and low-nutrient foods are plentiful, inexpensive, and widely available. Viewed as quick and cheap, such foods are attractive to families facing time and money pressures. And with so many media messages encouraging unhealthy eating, children and adolescents may have more negative than positive influences on their eating behavior. Too often, "healthy eating" carries images of expensive and tasteless food that is time-consuming to prepare.

Negative images also create barriers to physical activity: Regular physical activity is sometimes viewed as time-consuming, painful, boring, or expensive. Some people feel they can't keep up with regular physical activity, so they don't try any activity at all. People who are sedentary often feel that physical activity goals are beyond their reach, and others feel intimidated about joining in activities with others who are more athletic. Furthermore, some people have difficulty finding safe, inexpensive places where they can enjoy physical activity.

Improving the well-being of infants, children, and adolescents requires that health professionals, families, and communities work together to create opportunities for healthy eating and physical activity. Multifaceted, communitywide efforts are needed to combat negative images and to demonstrate that healthy eating can be quick and delicious and that physical activity can be fun. Using creative settings—such as community centers,

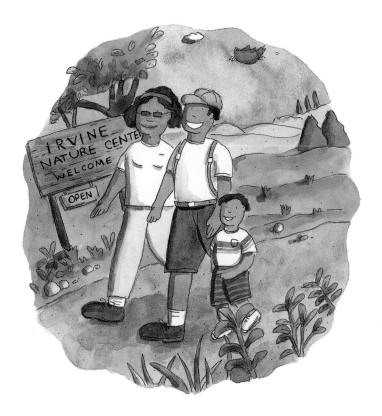

athletic facilities, libraries, restaurants, and supermarkets—to deliver innovative nutrition education programs should be explored. Environments that make it easier to be physically active—such as parks with play areas, walking and biking paths, and school and other community recreational facilities that are open after school and in the evenings—should be provided and maintained.

Healthy Eating

The food choices people make depend not only on their nutrition needs but also on their culture, access to food, environment, and enjoyment of certain foods. Eating is one of life's greatest pleasures, and a variety of factors play a role in how people select foods and plan meals.

To help children, adolescents, and families practice healthy eating behaviors and become more knowledgeable about the types and amounts of foods needed for optimal nutrition, the federal government created the following tools: the Dietary Guidelines for Americans, the Food Guide Pyramid, and the Nutrition Facts food label.[1-3] The Dietary Guidelines provide general nutrition principles, the Food Guide Pyramid shows how to select different types of foods for optimal nutrition, and the Nutrition Facts label identifies the nutrients in different food products. These tools can be used for children ages 2 and older and for adolescents.

Dietary Guidelines for Americans

The Dietary Guidelines are designed to help people choose foods that meet nutrition requirements, promote health, and support active lifestyles.

Food Guide Pyramid

The Food Guide Pyramid translates the Dietary Guidelines into food groups, listing the number of recommended daily servings from each group.

Figure 1. Food Guide Pyramid

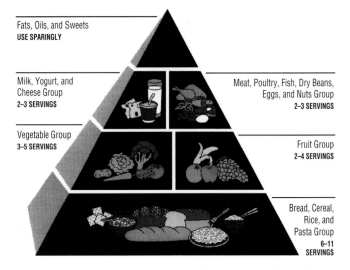

Note: A range of servings is given for each food group. The smaller number indicates the recommended servings for people who consume about 1,600 calories a day; the larger number indicates servings for people who consume about 2,800 calories a day.

Source: Dietary Guidelines Advisory Committee.[1]

Many children and adolescents from diverse cultures learn about nutrition in school by studying the Food Guide Pyramid. It is important to encourage children, adolescents, and families to maintain the healthy eating behaviors inherent in their cultures. Health professionals can make the Food Guide Pyramid relevant to different cultural groups by helping people place their traditional foods in the appropriate place in the pyramid. If traditional foods are at the top of the pyramid (and thus should be eaten sparingly), the frequency or amount of consumption may need to be changed, but few foods need to be eliminated completely.[4]

Figure 2. Food Guide Pyramid for Young Children

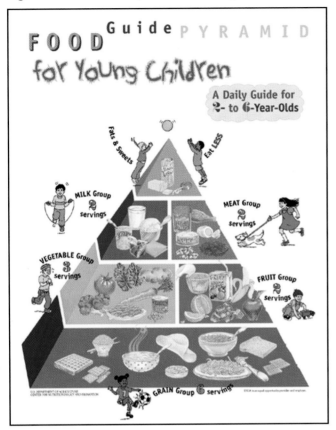

Source: U.S. Department of Agriculture, Center for Nutrition Policy and Promotion.[2]

The Food Guide Pyramid for Young Children was developed to help improve the diets of children ages 2 to 6. Although this adaptation of the original Food Guide Pyramid was needed because young children have unique eating behaviors and needs, the basic nutritional advice was not changed. As with the original pyramid, most of the daily servings of food should be selected from the food groups closest to the base of the pyramid. However, the Food Guide Pyramid for Young Children uses shorter food-group names and single numbers rather than ranges to indicate the recommended daily servings. The pyramid was designed to be more understandable and appealing to young children. In addition, illustrations of young children playing around the pyramid send the message that physical activity is important.

SERVING SIZES FOR CHILDREN AND ADOLESCENTS

Bread, Cereal, Rice, and Pasta Group
1 slice of bread
1 oz of ready-to-eat cereal
1/2 cup of cooked cereal
1/2 cup of rice or pasta

Vegetable Group
1 cup of raw, leafy vegetables
1/2 cup of raw or cooked vegetables
3/4 cup of vegetable juice

Fruit Group
1 medium apple, banana, or orange
1/2 cup of chopped, cooked, or canned fruit
3/4 cup of fruit juice
1/4 cup of dried fruit

Milk, Yogurt, and Cheese Group
1 cup of milk or yogurt
1 1/2 oz of natural cheese
2 oz of processed cheese

Meat, Poultry, Fish, Dry Beans, Eggs, and Nuts Group
2 to 3 oz of cooked lean meat, poultry, or fish
1/2 cup of cooked dry beans or 1 egg counts as 1 oz of lean meat. Two tablespoons of peanut butter or 1/3 cup of nuts counts as 1 oz of meat.

Offer children 2 to 3 years old about 2/3 of a serving, except for milk. Children 4 years and older and adolescents can eat these serving sizes. Children 2 to 6 years old need a total of 2 servings from the milk group each day.

Source: Dietary Guidelines Advisory Committee[1] and U.S. Department of Agriculture, Center for Nutrition Policy and Promotion.[2]

Nutrition Facts Label

The Nutrition Facts label helps people select foods that meet the Dietary Guidelines for Americans. The label provides a basis for comparing nutrients so that people can make informed choices when purchasing food products. The nutrition information on the label is based on a single serving, which reflects the amount a person typically eats at one time. Key nutrients, including total fat, cholesterol, sodium, potassium, total carbohydrate, and protein, are listed for each serving. The information is given as a percentage of Daily Values (DVs). This number shows how a serving of a specific food fits into a 2,000- or 2,500-calorie-a-day diet. The label also lists ingredients in descending order.[3]

Basic Principles of a Healthy Diet

Variety

Because no single food supplies all nutrients, a healthy diet needs to include a variety of foods from the Food Guide Pyramid's five major food groups. To meet nutrition recommendations, meals need to include grain products (i.e., bread, cereal, rice, pasta) accompanied by other vegetables, fruits, and low-fat selections from the remaining groups.[5]

Balance

A balanced diet incorporates appropriate amounts of foods from the five major food groups every day. Age, sex, and level of physical activity make a difference in the number of servings needed to maintain a well-balanced diet. People can maintain or improve their weight by balancing what they eat with regular physical activity.[5]

Moderation

Eating healthy foods helps promote nutritional status while controlling the intake of calories, as well as fat, saturated fat, cholesterol, salt, and sugar. Eating healthy foods in moderation allows people to enjoy the variety of foods available.[5]

Figure 3. Nutrition Facts

Macaroni and Cheese

Nutrition Facts

Serving Size 1 cup (228g)
Servings Per Container 2

Amount Per Serving

Calories 250   Calories from Fat 110

	% Daily Value*
Total Fat 12g	**18%**
Saturated Fat 3g	**15%**
Cholesterol 30mg	**10%**
Sodium 470mg	**20%**
Total Carbohydrate 31g	**10%**
Dietary Fiber 0g	**0%**
Sugars 5g	
Protein 5g	

Vitamin A	4%
Vitamin C	2%
Calcium	20%
Iron	4%

*Percent Daily Values are based on a 2,000 calorie diet. Your Daily Values may be higher or lower depending on your calorie needs:

	Calories:	2,000	2,500
Total Fat	Less than	65g	80g
Sat Fat	Less than	20g	25g
Cholesterol	Less than	300mg	300mg
Sodium		2,400mg	2,400mg
Total Carbohydrate		300g	375g
Dietary Fiber		25g	30g

Source: U.S. Department of Agriculture and U.S. Department of Health and Human Services.[3]

30 PERCENT FAT INTAKE AT DIFFERENT LEVELS OF CALORIC INTAKE

Calories	1,600	2,200	2,800
Total fat (grams)	53	73	93

Limiting Fat Intake

The Dietary Guidelines recommend that people limit fat intake to 30 percent or less of their total calories. Total grams of fat are determined in proportion to the recommended number of calories a person needs.

The following suggestions may help people limit their consumption of fat:

- Limit the consumption of high-fat sauces, salad dressings, and spreads (e.g, butter, margarine).
- Trim visible fat from meat.
- Limit the consumption of fried foods.
- Choose low-fat foods when eating at fast-food and other restaurants: Order low-fat milk instead of a shake, a single hamburger patty instead of two, or a salad instead of French fries.
- Have fruits and vegetables, rather than chips, cookies, and pastries, available for snacks.
- Use low-fat cooking methods such as baking, boiling, and broiling, and use cooking spray instead of oil, butter, shortening, or lard.

Limiting Sugar Intake

The following suggestions may help people limit their consumption of sugar:

- Eat foods that are naturally sweet, such as fresh fruits.
- Keep the sugar bowl off the table.
- Limit the consumption of heavily sweetened foods such as cookies and candy.
- Drink water, rather than fruit drinks or soft drinks, to quench thirst.

- Use less sugar and other sweeteners when cooking.
- Take along nutritious low-sugar snacks on outings.
- Develop a neighborhood policy on acceptable snacks for children and adolescents.

Nutrition Counseling

Health professionals can use the following information to help families promote healthy attitudes toward food and healthy eating behaviors.

Infancy

■ Infants have special dietary needs because of their rapid growth and development.

■ Breastmilk is the ideal food for infants. Even if the infant is breastfed for only a few weeks or months, the benefits are immeasurable.

■ Until the infant is 12 months of age, breastmilk or iron-fortified formula is recommended. Low-iron milk (e.g., cow's, goat's, soy) should not be used, even in infant cereal. Two percent, low-fat, and skim milk are not recommended during the first 2 years of life.

■ At about 4 to 6 months of age, when the infant is developmentally ready (i.e., infant is able to sit with support and has good control of the head and neck), supplemental foods can be introduced one at a time, at intervals of 7 days or more.

■ After the infant accepts iron-fortified infant cereal, fruits and vegetables can be offered. Fruits and vegetables rich in vitamin C help the infant absorb iron.

■ After the infant has eaten several varieties of fruits and vegetables, plain, soft meats such as well-cooked strained or pureed lean beef, pork, chicken, and turkey can be offered.

Early Childhood

- Calorie, fat, and cholesterol intake should not be restricted for children younger than 2 because this is a period of rapid growth and development, with high energy and nutrient requirements.

- After 2 years of age, children's diets need to gradually change so that, by the time they reach 5 years of age, they consume no more than 30 percent of their daily calories from fat.

- As children begin to consume fewer calories from fat, they need to eat more grain products; fruits; vegetables; low-fat milk products and other calcium-rich foods; and beans, lean meat, poultry, fish, and other protein-rich foods.

- Children 2 to 3 years of age need the same number of servings as children 4 to 6, but may need smaller portions, about two-thirds of a serving.

- Children 2 to 6 years of age need a total of two servings per day from the milk group.

- Children usually need three meals a day plus snacks.

- Because young children often eat small amounts of food at one time, offer nutritious foods (e.g., milk, fruit juices, fruits, vegetables, cooked meat or poultry, whole-grain crackers) as snacks.

Middle Childhood

- Caloric requirements vary during middle childhood. Children in this developmental period should be encouraged to eat at least the minimum number of recommended daily servings from each of the five major food groups every day.

- Consumption of high-fat and high-sugar foods at the top of the Food Guide Pyramid (e.g., butter, margarine, salad dressing, candy, soft drinks) should be limited.

Adolescence

- Adolescent males and physically active adolescent females need to eat the maximum number of recommended daily servings from each of the five major

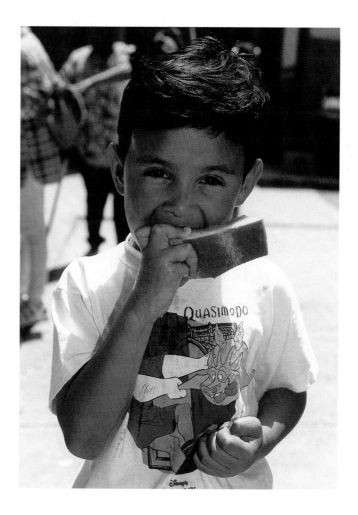

food groups every day. Most adolescent females need the middle ranges of servings, especially when they are active or growing.

- Adolescents need three servings per day from the milk, yogurt, and cheese group to meet their calcium needs, because bone density increases well into young adulthood (the 20s). Eating foods that provide enough calcium to attain maximum bone density helps prevent osteoporosis and bone fractures later in life.

Physical Activity

Regular physical activity in childhood and adolescence has many benefits: It improves strength and endurance, builds healthy bones and muscles, develops motor skills and coordination, controls weight, builds lean muscle, reduces fat, reduces feelings of depression and anxiety, and promotes psychological well-being.[6] In addition, many children and adolescents like physical activity because it is fun, they can do it with friends, and it helps them learn skills, stay in shape, and feel better.

Physical activity is any movement that uses energy. Physical activity encompasses a wide range of activities, from running, biking, swimming, and skating to walking, jumping rope, dancing, and playing group sports such as soccer, basketball, and volleyball.

The Surgeon General's report on physical activity recommends a moderate amount of daily physical activity for people of all ages. This goal can be achieved in long sessions of moderately intense activities, such as brisk walking for 30 minutes, or in short sessions of more intense activities, such as jogging or playing basketball for 15 to 20 minutes.[6]

To help people better understand new physical activity recommendations, the Activity Pyramid was developed. Similar to the federal government's Food Guide Pyramid, the Activity Pyramid illustrates a "balanced diet" of weekly physical activity and various forms of traditional exercise.[7]

Figure 4. Activity Pyramid

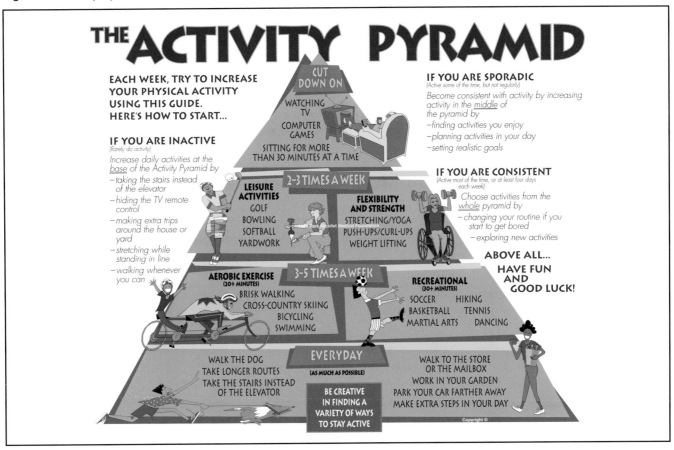

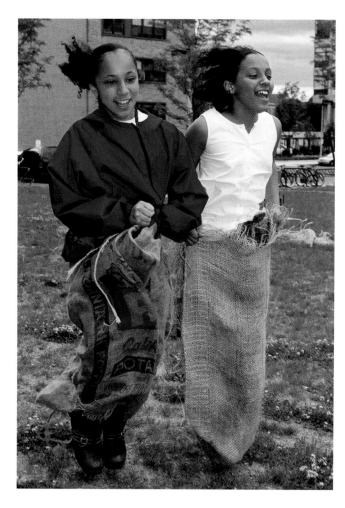

Some important principles of physical activity for children and adolescents follow.[8]

■ Children and adolescents are inherently active.

■ Children and adolescents have a relatively short attention span. However, with each passing year, they increase the length of time they can maintain interest in a specific activity.

■ Children and adolescents are concrete thinkers rather than abstract thinkers. They need concrete reasons for participating in an activity. If the reasons are too abstract, such as ensuring future health, they are unlikely to continue the activity.

■ Children and adolescents are active intermittently and need frequent rest periods.

■ Children and adolescents master their environment by learning to perform physical tasks.

■ Most children and adolescents learn physical activity skills during the school years.

■ Children and adolescents who are inactive are much more likely to be sedentary as adults.

■ Self-efficacy in physical activity is one of the best ways to ensure that children and adolescents will participate in physical activity throughout life.

■ Children and adolescents who have active families and who engage in regular physical activity with family members are more likely to be active than those whose families are not physically active.

■ Just as children and adolescents can get in the habit of participating in regular physical activity, they can also learn to be inactive if they are not given opportunities to be active.

■ Partnerships among health professionals, families, and communities can help children, adolescents, and their families adopt healthier lifestyles.

Physical Activity Counseling

Children and adolescents learn by example—if parents enjoy and participate in regular physical activity, their children and adolescents will too. Following are some ideas health professionals can share with children, adolescents, families, school personnel, and communities to encourage children and adolescents to participate in physical activity.

Tips for Families on Getting Started

■ Schedule time for physical activity.

■ Take turns selecting a physical activity the family can do together.

■ Buy toys and equipment that promote physical activity.

■ Buy fitness-oriented gifts.

■ Adapt activities to children and adolescents with special health care needs.

- Include grandparents, other relatives, and friends in physical activities.
- Help all family members find a physical activity that makes them feel good.
- Teach children and adolescents to play safely (e.g., by playing away from the street and wearing a helmet when biking).
- Emphasize the importance of having fun.

Tips for Promoting Physical Activity at Home

For Children and Adolescents

- Play indoor games.
- Jump rope.
- Walk a dog.
- Dance to music.
- Help with household chores—wash the floor, vacuum, mow the lawn, or sweep the walk.
- Build an obstacle course or fort.
- Rake leaves, then jump in them.

For Parents

- Limit the time that children and adolescents spend watching TV and videotapes and playing computer games to 1 to 2 hours a day.
- Identify safe places in the home where children can play.

Tips for Promoting Physical Activity at School

For School Personnel

- Provide children and adolescents with a mix of competitive team sports and noncompetitive activities.
- Encourage children and adolescents to play physically active games or sports during recess or break times.
- Set goals for increasing children's and adolescents' physical activity levels, and keep track of their progress.

- Provide protective clothing and proper equipment to prevent injuries.
- Offer health and physical education courses.
- Provide water for children and adolescents to drink while they participate in physical activity.

For Parents

- Talk to the physical education teacher about your child's or adolescent's physical education program and how you can provide support.
- Volunteer to help with physical activity events at your child's or adolescent's school.
- Encourage the physical education teacher to coordinate evening and weekend activities at school.
- Make sure that physical education teachers do not use physical activity as a punishment.
- Help organize an after-school recreation program.
- Encourage your child's or adolescent's school to offer opportunities for participating in physical activity every day.

Tips for Promoting Physical Activity in the Community

For Communities

- Provide children and adolescents with opportunities to participate in physical activities.
- Provide walking and biking areas.
- Encourage children and adolescents to participate in organized walks, runs, and bike-a-thons.
- Provide areas and equipment for water sports, such as canoeing and rafting.
- Offer classes in karate, ballet, and other physical activities.
- Provide safe areas for physical activity (e.g., biking, hiking, skating).

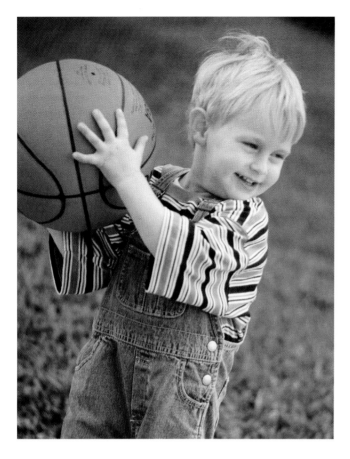

For Parents

■ Adopt a highway, park, or beach, and keep it clean.

■ Organize a family outing that includes physical activities.

■ Design play areas where climbing, jumping, and tumbling are allowed.

■ Identify safe places for children and adolescents to play and participate in physical activities.

■ Find free or low-cost physical activity areas, such as parks, walking and hiking trails, tennis courts, and community swimming pools.

■ Work with the community to ensure that children and adolescents from families with low incomes have transportation to and from physical activity programs and appropriate equipment.

References

1. Dietary Guidelines Advisory Committee. 2000. *Report of the Dietary Guidelines Advisory Committee on Dietary Guidelines for Americans, 2000.* Manuscript in preparation. Available from http://www.ars.usda.gov/dgac/.

2. U.S. Department of Agriculture, Center for Nutrition Policy and Promotion. 1999. *Tips for Using the Food Guide Pyramid for Young Children 2 to 6 Years Old.* Washington, DC: U.S. Department of Agriculture, Center for Nutrition Policy and Promotion.

3. U.S. Department of Health and Human Services, Food and Drug Administration. 1996. *The Food Label and You: Check It Out!* Rockville, MD: U.S. Department of Health and Human Services, Food and Drug Administration.

4. Shaw A, Fulton L, Davis C, Hogbin M. 1996. *Using the Food Guide Pyramid: A Resource for Nutrition Educators.* Washington, DC: U.S. Department of Agriculture, Center for Nutrition Policy and Promotion.

5. International Food Information Council Foundation, U.S. Department of Agriculture, and Food Marketing Institute. 1996. *The Food Guide Pyramid: Your Personal Guide to Healthful Eating.* Washington, DC: International Food Information Council Foundation, U.S. Department of Agriculture, and Food Marketing Institute.

6. Centers for Disease Control and Prevention, National Center for Chronic Disease Prevention and Health Promotion, and President's Council on Physical Fitness and Sports. 1996. *Physical Activity and Health: A Report of the Surgeon General.* Washington, DC: Centers for Disease Control and Prevention, National Center for Chronic Disease Prevention and Health Promotion, and President's Council on Physical Fitness and Sports.

7. Institute for Research and Education HealthSystem Minnesota, Health Education Center. 1996. *Building Your Activity Pyramid.* Minneapolis, MN: Institute for Research and Education HealthSystem Minnesota, Health Education Center.

8. Corbin CB, Pangrazi RP. 1998. *Physical Activity for Children: A Statement of Guidelines.* Reston, VA: National Association for Sport and Physical Education.

CULTURAL AWARENESS IN NUTRITION COUNSELING

All people belong to some kind of cultural group. Culture influences the way people look at things, how they interact with others, and how they expect others to behave. Health professionals need to understand how their own cultures influence their attitudes and behaviors, and they need to understand other cultures and their implications for nutrition counseling.

Providing nutrition supervision to people from diverse cultural backgrounds can be both challenging and rewarding. Health professionals are given the opportunity to observe people and their traditions, including the foods they eat and occasions they celebrate. Such observations can enhance the health professional's awareness and knowledge of other cultures.

Culture and Food

Food choices, which can be very personal, are influenced by culture. For many people, culture-specific foods are closely linked to their families and strong feelings of being cared for and nurtured. However, when discussing their food choices, people may respond by saying what they think the health professional wants to hear. Health professionals can encourage people to be more candid by asking open-ended, nonjudgmental questions.

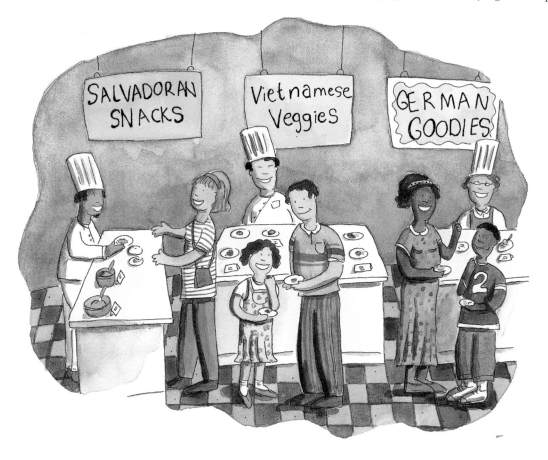

The role of certain foods varies among cultures, but in most cultures, food is used for similar purposes. For example, in all cultures, staple, or core, foods form the foundation of the diet. A staple food—such as rice or beans—is typically bland, relatively inexpensive, easy to prepare, an important source of calories, and an indispensable part of the diet. In addition, people from virtually all cultures use food during celebrations, and many use food as medicine or to promote health.

Culture also influences how people prepare food, how they use seasonings, and how often they eat certain foods. These behaviors can differ from region to region and from family to family.

Acculturation—the adoption of the beliefs, values, attitudes, and behaviors of a dominant, or mainstream, culture—also influences a person's food choices. Acculturation may involve altering traditional eating behaviors to make them similar to those of the dominant culture. These changes can be grouped into three categories: (1) the addition of new foods, (2) the substitution of foods, and (3) the rejection of foods. People add new foods to their diets for several reasons, including increased economic status and food availability (especially if the food is not readily available in the person's homeland). Substitution may occur because new foods are more convenient to prepare, more affordable, or better liked than traditional ones. People, particularly children and adolescents, may reject eating traditional foods because it make them feel different.

Keys to Good Cross-Cultural Communication

Good communication during nutrition supervision is important for providing anticipatory guidance. To keep the lines of communication open, health professionals must overcome any real or perceived differences between them and the people they serve. Being open, honest, respectful, nonjudgmental, and, most important, willing to listen and learn is critical. Health professionals can help people in a way that maintains their dignity. Some keys to good cross-cultural communication follow:[1]

- *Respect personal space.* Health professionals can make people feel comfortable by asking them to sit where they want. This allows people to have the personal space they need.

- *Learn and follow cultural rules about touching.* It is essential for health professionals to learn these rules, including rules based on a person's sex. For example, in some Asian cultures, a person's head should not be touched because the head is considered the "seat of wisdom." In some American Indian cultures, a vigorous handshake may be considered a sign of aggression.

- *Establish rapport.* Health professionals can establish rapport with people by sharing experiences, exchanging information, and greeting and responding to them in culturally appropriate ways.

- *Express interest in people.* Health professionals can express interest in various ways: by smiling, being friendly and warm, asking questions (even about things they are unfamiliar or uncomfortable with), showing respect, and demonstrating that they are open-minded and trustworthy. Paying attention to children is also a good idea: This may impress mothers from particular cultures. However, health professionals need to be aware that people from some cultures believe that it is inappropriate to accept compliments about their children, especially if the children are present.

- *Listen carefully.* Health professionals must listen carefully and not interrupt people or try to put words in their mouths.

- *Respect silence.* Health professionals do not have to fill a silent moment with small talk. People need a chance to gather their thoughts, especially when they are trying to speak in a language they are not familiar with.

- *Notice how people make eye contact.* Health professionals need to observe how people make eye contact with family members and others. Many cultures consider it impolite to look directly at the person who is speaking. Lowering the eyes and glancing sideways may be seen as respectful, especially if the speaker is older or in a position of authority.

- *Pay attention to body language.* Health professionals must learn what messages are conveyed by body movements, such as turning up the palms of the hands, waving, and pointing, and which gestures should be avoided.

- *Reach the appropriate family member.* In some cultures, the oldest male is considered the head of the family, while in others, an elderly female has this role. Health professionals must ensure that their messages reach the head of the family.

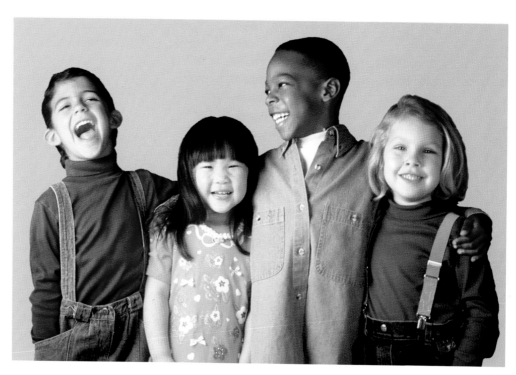

- *Study a person's responses.* A "yes" response does not necessarily indicate that a person understands the message or is willing to do what is being discussed. The person may simply be showing respect for the health professional. For example, American Indians may not ask questions because they believe this would indicate that the health professional was not communicating clearly. People may smile or laugh to mask emotions or prevent conflict. Health professionals can make sure that a person understands by asking questions.

Special Nutrition Concerns for Culturally Diverse Populations

Food and Health Beliefs

In many cultures, people believe that food promotes health, cures disease, or has other medicinal qualities. In addition, many people believe that maintaining balance is important to health. For example, traditional Chinese people maintain that health and disease are related to the balance between the "yin" and "yang" forces in the body. Diseases caused by yin forces are treated with yang foods to restore balance, and vice versa. In Puerto Rico, foods are classified as hot or cold (which may not reflect the temperature or spiciness of foods), and people believe that maintaining a balance between these two types of foods is important to health. Health professionals can become more effective by exploring such beliefs and incorporating them in their nutrition messages. (See *Ethnic and Regional Food Practices: A Series* in the list of suggested reading.)

Lactose Intolerance

Lactose intolerance is much more common in people of non-European ancestry. People who are lactose-intolerant may experience cramps and diarrhea when they eat moderate to large amounts of foods that contain lactose, such as milk and other dairy products. Children and adolescents may be able to avoid symptoms by consuming small servings of milk throughout the day or by consuming lactose-reduced milk or lactase tablets or drops with milk. Cheese and yogurt are often better tolerated than milk because they contain less lactose. For people who cannot tolerate any milk or dairy products in their diet, health professionals can suggest other sources of calcium, such as dark green, leafy vegetables; tofu or corn tortillas processed with calcium; and calcium-fortified orange juice.

Culturally Based Attitudes

People from different cultures may view body weight differently. Keeping a child from being underweight may be very important to people from cultures in which poverty or insufficient food supplies are common. They may view excess weight as healthy and might be offended if a health professional refers to their children as overweight.

Summary

To meet the challenge of providing nutrition supervision to diverse populations, health professionals must learn to respect and appreciate the variety of cultural traditions related to food and the wide variation in food practices within and among cultural groups. Health professionals can take advantage of interactions with people from other cultures by sharing food experiences, asking questions, observing the food choices people make, and working with the community.

Reference

1. Graves DE, Suitor CW. 1998. *Celebrating Diversity: Approaching Families through Their Food* (rev. ed.). Arlington, VA: National Center for Education in Maternal and Child Health.

Suggested Reading

American Diabetes Association and The American Dietetic Association. 1989–1996. *Ethnic and Regional Food Practices: A Series*. Chicago, IL: The American Dietetic Association.

Probert KL, ed. 1996. *Moving to the Future: Developing Community-Based Nutrition Services*. Washington, DC: Association of State and Territorial Public Health Nutrition Directors.

Probert KL. 1997. *Moving to the Future: Developing Community-Based Nutrition Services—Workbook and Training Manual*. Washington, DC: Association of State and Territorial Public Health Nutrition Directors.

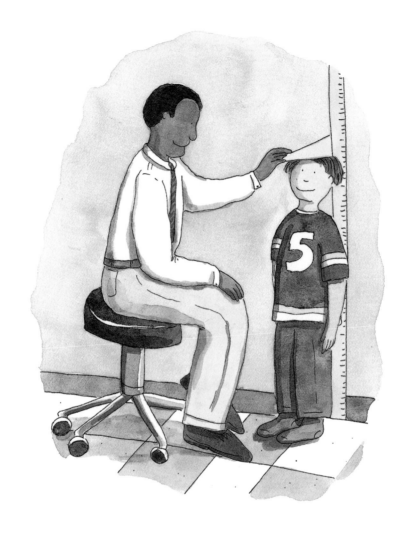

Nutrition
Supervision Guidelines

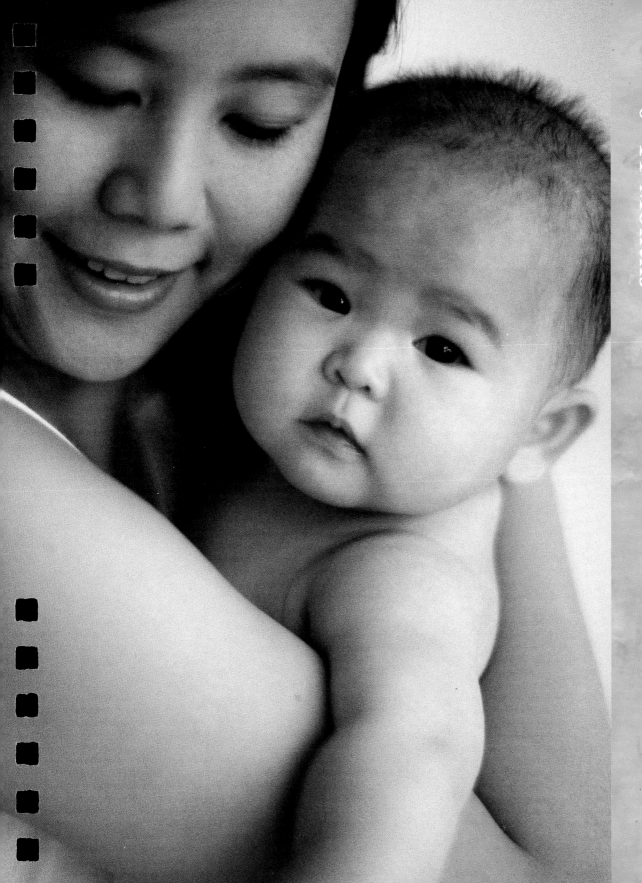

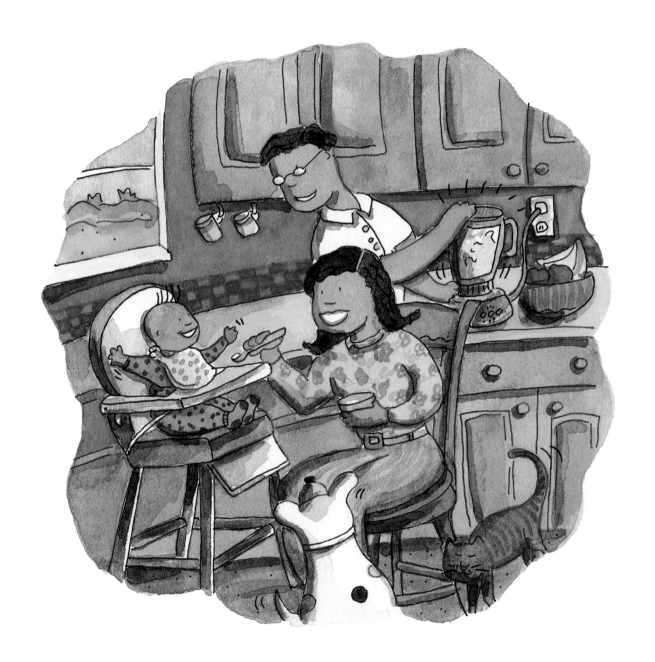

INFANCY

Infancy is a period marked by the most rapid physical growth and development of a person's life, and the energy required to support these processes is phenomenal. Infancy is divided into several stages, with physical growth, developmental achievements, nutrition needs, and feeding patterns varying significantly in each. The most rapid growth occurs in early infancy, between birth and 6 months of age. During the first 2 to 6 weeks of life, the infant eats, sleeps, and grows. In middle infancy, from 6 to 9 months, and late infancy, from 9 to 12 months, growth slows but is still rapid. In late infancy, infants' physical maturation, mastery of purposeful activity, and loss of newborn reflexes allow them to eat a wider variety of foods.[1]

Infants' vitality and successful development depend on good nutrition in the first year of life. Full-term infants who are fed on demand usually consume the amount they need to grow well. But feeding infants is much more complex than simply offering food when they are hungry, and it serves purposes far beyond supporting their physical growth. Feeding provides opportunities for emotional bonding between the parent and infant.

When feeding their infant, parents clarify and strengthen their sense of what it means to be a parent. They gain a sense of responsibility by caring for an infant, they experience frustration when they cannot interpret the infant's cues, and they further develop their ability to negotiate and solve problems through their interactions with the infant. They also identify their values and priorities, and expand their abilities to meet their infant's needs. Anticipatory guidance from health professionals can reinforce parents' strengths and encourage good parenting.

Growth and Physical Development

Immediately after birth, infants lose approximately 6 percent of their body weight because of fluid loss and some breakdown of tissue. Infants usually regain their birthweight by 10 to 14 days after birth, and thereafter weight gain proceeds at a slower rate. Typically, infants double their birthweight by 4 to 6 months and triple it by 1 year. On average, infants gain 5 to 7 oz per week in the first 4 to 6 months and 3 to 5 oz per week from 6 to 18 months. Infants usually increase their length by 50 percent in the first year, but the rate of increase slows down during the second half of the year. From birth to 6 months, infants gain approximately 1 inch a month, and from 6 to 12 months of age, they gain about $1/2$ inch each month.

Growth rates of breastfed and formula-fed infants differ. Breastfed infants grow more rapidly in the first 2 to 3 months but less rapidly from 3 to 12 months of age. Infants who are genetically determined to be tall but who are born short may experience catch-up growth during the first 3 to 6 months. However, infants who are genetically determined to be short but who are long at birth tend to maintain the same rate of growth for several months and then experience a lag down in growth.

To meet growth demands, infants require a high intake of calories as well as adequate intake of fat, protein, vitamins, and minerals. From birth to 6 months of age, infants require about 108 kcal/kg of body weight per day. By 12 months, this need decreases to 100 kcal/kg per day. Fats must constitute at least 30 percent of caloric intake to meet the demands of growth and development. Vitamin and mineral needs are usually met if the infant is breast-fed by a well-nourished mother or receives correctly prepared infant formula.

Significant developmental changes that occur in the first year have a profound effect on the way infants feed. Newborns are able to locate the mother's breast, latch onto the nipple, and suck to receive colostrum and then milk. At about 4 to 6 months of age, infants may be ready to eat soft, moist foods. Over the next few months, they will learn to chew and swallow, manipulate finger foods, drink from a cup, and ultimately feed themselves.

As infants grow, their ability to digest a greater volume and variety of foods increases. Thus, new-borns need small, frequent feedings, whereas older infants are able to consume more milk at one time and require fewer feedings. The digestive systems of newborns are designed to effectively digest breast-milk. By 6 months of age, an infant's digestive system has matured enough to allow the absorption of more complex foods.

For most infants, the first primary tooth appears around 6 months of age. Teeth erupt every few months, usually in right and left pairs alternating between the upper and lower jaws, and proceeding from the front of the mouth to the back. These first teeth, however, do not change how infants process food, because they usually gum their food even if they have teeth.

Infants 6 months and older need fluoride to protect the teeth. The risk of developing early child-hood caries can be reduced if infants at this age drink fluoridated water or take fluoride supplements. This is especially important if the water is severely deficient in fluoride (less than 0.3 ppm).[2]

Social and Emotional Development

Feeding is crucial for developing a healthy relationship between parents and infants. A parent's responsiveness to an infant's cues of hunger and satiation and the close physical contact during feeding facilitate healthy social and emotional development. During the first year, being fed when hungry helps infants develop the trust that their needs will be met. For optimum development, newborns need to be fed as soon as possible when they express hunger. As they grow older and become more secure in that trust, infants can wait longer for feeding.

Quickly responding to their infant's cues also strengthens parents' sense of competence. As they feed their infant, they learn how their actions comfort and satisfy. Over time, parents become more skilled at interpreting their infant's cues, and they increase their repertoire of successful responses to those cues. Physical contact during feeding enhances communication between the parent and infant because it provides the infant with essential sensory stimulation, including skin and eye contact, and strengthens the psychological bond between the parent and infant. A sense of caring and trust evolves and lays the groundwork for communication patterns throughout life.

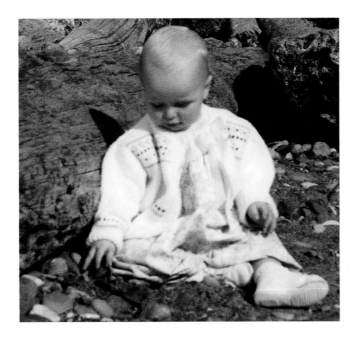

Healthy Lifestyles

During infancy, the amount and type of physical activity change dramatically. At first, infants spend most of their time sleeping and eating. Activity begins with reflexes that ensure the infant's survival. Over the next few months, these reflexes disappear, and infants slowly gain voluntary control over their movements. With increasing control comes more physical activity, including sitting up, rolling over, crawling, standing, and eventually walking.

Development is an individual process. Some infants sit earlier than others. Some walk as early as 9 months, and others walk months after their first birthday. Although the order in which infants acquire motor skills is the same, the speed with which they acquire them is individual. The ways infants are held and handled, the toys they play with, and their environment all influence their physical activity and motor skills development.

Families that play with their infants, encouraging rolling, crawling, and then walking, are nurturing this development.

Partnerships with the Community

Partnerships among health professionals, families, and communities are essential for ensuring that parents receive guidance on infant nutrition and feeding. Health professionals can have a tremendous impact on decisions about infant feeding as they inform parents about the various options for infant feeding. They provide an opportunity for parents to discuss, reflect on, and decide which options best suit their circumstances. Health professionals also identify and contact community resources that help parents.

Many hospitals, including those striving to meet the requirements of the World Health Organization and UNICEF Baby-Friendly Hospital Initiative, are taking the following steps to promote and support breastfeeding:

1. Developing a written breastfeeding policy and communicating it to all health care staff

2. Training staff members to ensure that they have the skills to implement the policy

3. Educating pregnant women about the benefits and management of breastfeeding

4. Initiating breastfeeding early

5. Educating mothers on how to breastfeed and maintain lactation

6. Limiting the use of any foods or beverages other than breastmilk

7. Having newborns stay in the mother's room

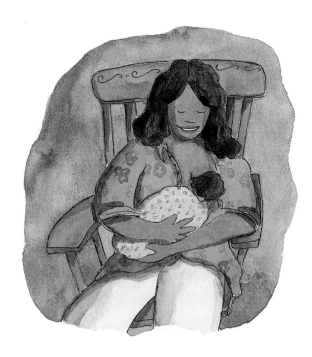

8. Supporting mothers so that they can breastfeed their infants on demand

9. Limiting the use of pacifiers

10. Fostering breastfeeding support groups[3]

Health professionals should be aware of lactation specialists available in the area and tell parents about the benefits of using these specialists, even for mothers who have breastfed before. In many cases, lactation specialists provide follow-up care after the mother and infant are discharged from the hospital, consult with the mother by phone, and schedule follow-up visits in a hospital-based lactation clinic. They also offer suggestions to health professionals for use during follow-up visits. Moreover, lactation specialists help families manage breastfeeding when mothers return to work or when breastfeeding needs to be interrupted because of severe illness in the mother or infant. Breastfeeding support groups, such as La Leche League, may be available in the community.

As more women breastfeed, some workplaces are adapting to meet their needs. Some employers offer longer breaks and a private setting for pumping breastmilk, refrigeration to safely store breastmilk, and on-site child care so that mothers can breastfeed their infants during the workday.

Other nutrition resources may be available in the community. For adolescent parents, school programs can focus on the importance of prenatal nutrition, the value and benefits of breastfeeding, and the nutrition needs of infants. Health departments offer similar educational services through WIC and other programs in which community health nurses or nutritionists visit families at home. Health maintenance organizations and community hospitals may also offer infant nutrition education.

The community may also need to supply financial resources to families to ensure that their infants are adequately nourished. For families with low incomes, WIC offers a food package for pregnant, postpartum, and breastfeeding women and for infants and children up to 5 years of age. Families may also qualify for programs such as the Food Stamp Program. (See Appendix K: Federal Food Assistance and Nutrition Programs.) A community food shelf or pantry can provide additional food for families in need. In some cases, infants may need access to human breastmilk banks. Families may also need assistance in procuring special equipment, such as breast pumps, special nipples, and bottles.

Common Nutrition Concerns

Many parents are concerned about whether to feed their infants breastmilk or infant formula. They want to be certain their infants are receiving the nutrients they need but are unsure whether breastfeeding or bottle feeding is best. Health professionals should emphasize that breastmilk is the ideal food for infants and encourage breastfeeding whenever possible.[4] Even if the infant is breastfed for only a few weeks or months, the benefits are innumerable. Health professionals can help identify barriers to breastfeeding and provide referrals to lactation support services. For infants with special health care needs, breastfeeding can be successful, although mothers may need extra emotional support, instruction about special techniques for positioning, or special equipment to help overcome feeding problems.

Health professionals can help families decide when to introduce supplemental foods into the infant's diet by providing information on the infant's nutrition needs and developmental abilities. Infants are developmentally ready to eat supplemental foods by about 4 to 6 months, when their sucking reflex has changed to allow coordinated swallowing, they can sit with support, and they have good head and neck control. Cognitively, infants begin to associate feeding with satiation and comfort and are able to cooperate during feeding. Between 6 and 12 months, infants master chewing, swallowing, and manipulation of finger foods; begin to use cups and utensils; and try foods with different tastes and textures.

Infants with special health care needs may have feeding challenges. Resources are available to provide education and support for parents of infants with these needs. For infants with developmental disabilities, nutrition problems may be addressed as part of nutrition therapy in an early intervention program. (See the Children and Adolescents with Special Health Care Needs chapter.)

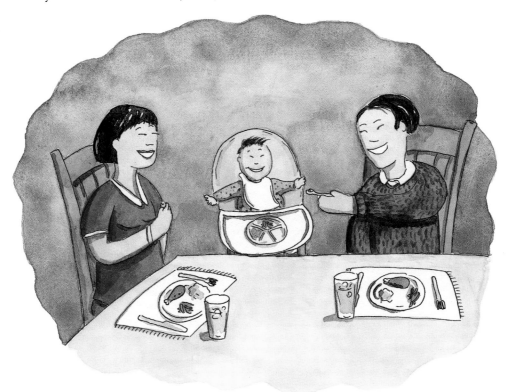

INFANCY NUTRITION SUPERVISION

An infant's nutrition status should be evaluated during comprehensive nutrition supervision visits or as part of general health supervision visits. (For more information on health supervision, see *Bright Futures: Guidelines for Health Supervision of Infants, Children, and Adolescents*, listed under Suggested Reading in this chapter.)

Health professionals begin nutrition supervision by gathering information about the infant's nutrition status. This can be accomplished by selectively asking key interview questions listed in this chapter or by reviewing a questionnaire filled out by parents before the visit. (See Appendix A: Nutrition Questionnaire for Infants.) These methods provide a useful starting point for identifying nutrition concerns.

Health professionals can then use this chapter's screening and assessment guidelines, and nutrition counseling guidelines, to provide families with anticipatory guidance. Nutrition supervision information that pertains to the entire infancy developmental period (Nutrition Supervision Throughout Infancy) is provided first in this chapter, followed by information for age-specific visits. Interview questions, screening and assessment, and nutrition counseling should be used as appropriate and will vary from visit to visit and from infant to infant.

To assist health professionals in promoting optimal nutrition that will last a lifetime, desired outcomes for the infant and responsibilities for the family are identified in Table 1.

Nutrition Supervision Throughout Infancy

Interview Questions

Health professionals can ask the following questions to elicit key nutrition information:

How do you think feeding is going? Do you have any questions about breastfeeding Shelley?

How does Shelley let you know when she is hungry? How do you know when she has had enough to eat?

How often is Shelley eating?

Have you noticed changes in the way she eats?

How do you feel about the way Shelley is growing?

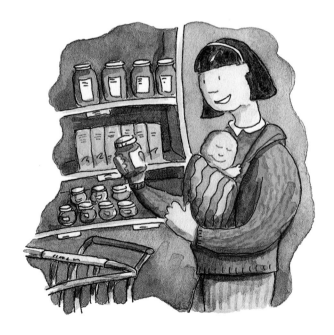

Are you concerned about having enough money to buy food or infant formula?

What is the source of your drinking and cooking water? Do you use bottled or processed water?

Do you smoke? Does anyone smoke in your house?

Screening and Assessment

■ Measure the infant's length, weight, and head circumference, and plot these on a standard growth chart (e.g., the revised Centers for Disease Control and Prevention [CDC]/National Center for Health Statistics [NCHS] growth chart). Deviation from the expected growth pattern (e.g., a major change in growth percentiles on the chart) should be evaluated. This may be normal or may indicate a nutrition problem (e.g., difficulties with eating).

■ Evaluate the appearance of the infant's skin, hair, teeth, gums, tongue, and eyes.

■ Observe the parent-infant interaction and assess their responses to one another (e.g., affectionate, comfortable, distant, anxious).

Nutrition Counseling

Health professionals can use the following information to provide anticipatory guidance to parents. Anticipatory guidance provides information on the infant's nutrition status and on what to expect as the infant enters the next developmental period, and fosters the promotion of healthy eating behaviors. (For additional information on nutrition counseling, see Appendix G: Strategies for Health Professionals to Promote Healthy Eating Behaviors.)

For Parents of All Infants

■ Explain to parents that preterm or low-birth-weight infants younger than 6 months who are breastfed or who are not fed an iron-fortified formula may need iron supplements. Because these infants are born with much less stored iron than full-term infants and experience a greater rate of growth during infancy, their iron stores become depleted much earlier, often by 2 to 3 months of age. Iron-deficiency anemia should be confirmed or ruled out by subsequent measurement of hemoglobin and hematocrit based on capillary blood sampling. After diagnosis, iron-deficiency anemia can be treated with oral (elemental) iron, at 3 mg/kg per day for 4 weeks.[5]

■ Although clinical vitamin B_{12} deficiency is rare, a breastfed infant may need vitamin B_{12} supplements before 6 months of age if the mother is vitamin B_{12} deficient (e.g., if she is a vegan [eats no animal products], if she is undernourished and does not take B_{12} supplements).

■ Vitamin D supplements may be needed if the infant is not exposed to adequate sunlight, especially if the infant has very dark skin or is living in areas with limited sunlight.[4]

■ Emphasize to parents that an infant weaned from breastmilk before 12 months needs iron-fortified infant formula rather than cow's milk.[4]

■ Until the infant is 12 months, breastmilk or iron-fortified infant formula is recommended and low-iron milk (e.g., cow's, goat's, soy) should not be used, even in infant cereal.[6]

■ Inform parents that the infant needs fat for growth and energy and that they should not restrict the infant's fat intake. Between 2 and 6 months of age, body fat increases twice as much as muscle; therefore, many infants seem chubby at 6 months. Girls deposit a greater percentage of fat than boys. Between 6 and 12 months, however, infants gain more muscle and less fat, and the chubby appearance often disappears.

■ Reassure parents that it is normal for infants to spit up a little milk at each feeding. Burping the infant several times during a feeding, and avoiding excessive movement soon after a feeding, may help.

■ Explain to parents that infants who are constipated (i.e., who have hard, dry stools that are passed with difficulty) may not be getting enough breastmilk or infant formula, may be receiving formula that is prepared incorrectly, or may be eating other foods too soon. Constipation is uncommon in breastfed infants, although breastfed infants 6 weeks and older may go several days without a bowel movement.

■ Explain to parents that infants who have diarrhea, fever, or other illnesses may need to drink extra water or other fluids as directed by a health professional.

■ Tell parents to discard any bottles of expressed breastmilk or open containers of ready-to-feed or concentrated infant formula that have been stored in the refrigerator for 48 hours or more. Any bottles of prepared infant formula stored in the refrigerator should be discarded after 24 hours.[7]

■ Tell parents not to warm expressed breastmilk, infant formula, or any food in containers or jars in a microwave. The container may feel cool, but the contents can be too hot because of uneven heating and cause a burn.[7] Bottles can be warmed by holding them under hot running water or placing them in a bowl of hot water for a few minutes. To make sure that the fluid isn't too warm, parents can sprinkle a few drops on their wrist (it should feel lukewarm). If necessary, they can wait for it to cool down and test it again.

■ Reassure parents that infants develop feeding skills at their own rates. The infant must be ready before being introduced to new foods and textures. If the infant has significant delays in the development of feeding skills, further assessment by a health professional is needed.

■ Emphasize that choking can be a problem for infants because they may not have enough muscle control to chew and swallow foods properly. Infants can choke on foods that are small or slippery (e.g., hard candy, whole grapes, hot dogs) and foods that are dry and difficult to chew (e.g., popcorn, raw carrots, nuts). Foods that are sticky or tough to break apart (e.g., peanut butter, large chunks of meat) can get lodged in the throat.[7]

■ Tell parents not to add honey to food, water, or formula because it can be a source of spores that cause botulism poisoning in infants. Processed foods containing honey should not be given to infants.[6]

■ Inform parents that infants are at high risk for many foodborne illnesses because their immune and gastrointestinal systems are not fully devel-

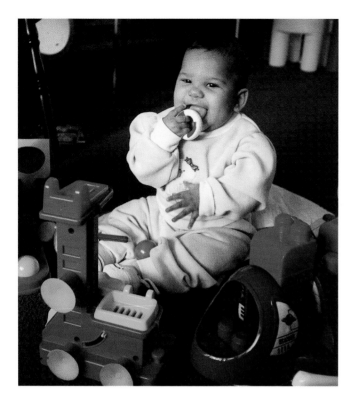

oped. To reduce the risk of foodborne illness, parents need to follow food safety practices. (See Appendix H: Tips for Promoting Food Safety.)

■ Instruct parents to clean the infant's gums and teeth twice a day. A clean, moist washcloth can be used to wipe the gums. A small, soft toothbrush (without toothpaste) and water can be used to clean the teeth.

■ Explain to parents that early childhood caries (baby bottle tooth decay) may result from frequent or prolonged bottle feedings or snacking on sugary or carbohydrate-rich foods. Giving infants a bottle filled with anything but water to encourage sleep or to quiet them may promote caries in newly erupted primary teeth if decay-causing bacteria are present in the mouth. To

help prevent early childhood caries, parents should introduce a cup for drinking at 6 months and wean their infant from the bottle by 12 to 14 months. Juice should be provided in a cup instead of a bottle and limited to 4 oz per day.

■ Explain to parents that community water fluoridation is a safe and effective way to significantly reduce the risk of early childhood caries in infants. It is best for families to drink fluoridated water; for families that prefer bottled water, a brand in which fluoride is added at a concentration of approximately 0.8 to 1.0 mg/L (ppm) is recommended.[2]

■ Inform parents that infants 6 months and older who receive breastmilk or infant formula prepared with water require fluoride supplementation if the water is severely deficient in fluoride (less than 0.3 ppm).[2]

■ Inform parents that they can prevent infant injury by using a safety belt when the infant is placed in a shopping cart.

■ Explain to parents that long-term exposure to secondhand smoke may put infants at risk for respiratory illness and heart disease. Tell parents not to smoke or allow others to smoke in their home. If parents do smoke, they should avoid smoking in the car, inside the home, or anywhere near infants.[8]

For Mothers of Breastfed Infants

■ Breastfeeding an infant exclusively for about the first 6 months of life provides ideal nutrition and supports the best possible growth and development.[4]

■ Inform parents that breastfeeding can continue for 12 months or as long as the mother and infant wish to continue.[4]

■ Explain that breastfeeding can be more relaxing if the mother has a quiet place to breastfeed. The feeding position should be comfortable and the experience nurturing for the infant.

■ Encourage fathers to help care for breastfed infants. Fathers can bring the infant to the mother when it is time to breastfeed. When the infant is finished breastfeeding, the father can cuddle the infant and help with burping, diapering, or bathing.

■ Explain to parents that the longer an infant sucks, the more breastmilk the mother's body will make. Feeding the infant on demand is the best way to stimulate the lactation process. Manually expressing milk or using a breast pump is recommended to increase or maintain milk supply when the mother is away from her infant.

■ Emphasize that the infant should be allowed to finish feeding at one breast before the other breast is offered. The length of feedings should not be restricted, although 20 to 45 minutes provides adequate intake and allows the mother some time to rest between feedings.

■ Inform parents that the frequency of feedings is typically 8 to 12 times in 24 hours. In the first 2 to 4 weeks, infants should not be allowed to sleep more than 4 hours without breastfeeding.

■ Explain that infants have periods when they grow very fast. At these times, it may be necessary to feed them more often to give the mother's milk production a chance to adjust to the infant's needs. Frequent feedings help establish

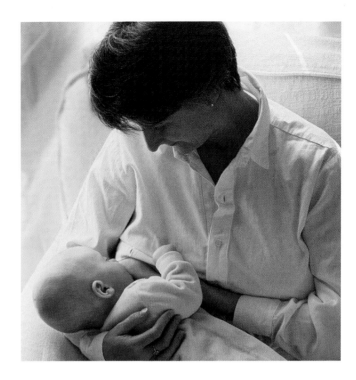

milk supply and prevent the breasts from getting too full.

■ Emphasize that mothers who are breastfeeding more than one infant may need to eat more, receive additional nutrition counseling, and have extra help at home.

■ Additional sources of breastfeeding information include friends and family, support groups (e.g., La Leche League), lactation consultants, and educational materials.

■ Tell parents to use refrigerated, expressed breastmilk within 48 hours. Safe storage time for frozen milk ranges from 2 weeks to 6 months, depending on the temperature in the freezer.[7]

■ Encourage mothers to eat a variety of healthy foods. Eating well helps the mother stay healthy and the infant grow. (See the Healthy Eating and Physical Activity chapter.)

- Encourage mothers to drink liquids such as milk or juice when they are thirsty and to drink a glass of water at every feeding.

- Tell mothers to limit the consumption of drinks containing caffeine (e.g., coffee, tea, soft drinks) to two servings per day.[9]

- Explain that it is best for the mother to avoid drinking alcoholic beverages. If she does, no more than 2 to 2 1/2 oz of liquor, 8 oz of wine, or 2 cans of beer should be consumed per day (less for small women).[9]

- Instruct parents to gradually introduce well-cooked, strained or pureed meats with iron (e.g., lean beef, pork, chicken, turkey) in the second half of the first year to supplement breastfeeding.[4]

For Parents of Formula-Fed Infants

- Explain to parents that iron-fortified infant formula is an appropriate substitute for breastmilk for feeding the full-term infant during the first year of life.

- Tell parents to carefully prepare infant formula as instructed and to follow these sanitary procedures:

    Wash their hands before preparing infant formula.

    Clean the area where infant formula is prepared.

    Clean and disinfect reusable bottles, caps, and nipples before every use.

    Wash and dry the top of the infant formula container before opening.

- Emphasize that cereal or other foods should not be added to formula.

- Tell parents to discard any milk left in the bottle when the infant has finished eating. A bottle that has been started should not be reused.

- Inform parents that open containers of ready-to-feed or concentrated infant formula should be covered and refrigerated.[7]

- Powdered infant formula can be stored at room temperature.

- Encourage parents to hold the infant close, in a semi-upright position, during feeding. The parent should be able to look into the infant's eyes.

- Discuss with parents that they will need to prepare and offer more infant formula as the infant's appetite increases.

- Inform parents that infants do not usually need water, but water can be offered on hot days between feedings.

- Instruct parents to check the following if the infant is crying more than usual or seems to want to eat all the time:

    Is the infant positioned in a semi-erect, comfortable position for feeding?

    Is the formula prepared correctly? Has too much water been added?

    Is the bottle nipple too firm? Is the nipple hole too large?

    Are they responding to the infant's cues of hunger?

    Is the feeding environment too distracting?

Nutrition Supervision by Visit

PRENATAL

Interview Questions

For Pregnant Women

Have you thought about breastfeeding?

Do you know about the benefits of breastfeeding for you and your baby?

Do you have any concerns about your diet and breastfeeding?

Do you restrict any foods in your diet because of lack of appetite, food aversions, vegan or vegetarian diets, weight gain, food allergies and sensitivities, or any other reason?

Does your family have a history of food allergies?

Are you taking prenatal vitamins? Do you plan to take any in the future?

Do you take any vitamin or mineral supplements?

Do you drink wine, beer, or other alcoholic beverages?

Do you use any drugs (for example, prescription, over-the-counter, or illegal)?

Do you have any questions about feeding your baby?

What experiences have you had feeding babies? With your own children? Other children? Your siblings?

What does your partner or family think about your plan for feeding?

Are you concerned about having enough money to buy food?

Do you smoke? Does anyone smoke in your home?

Do you have problems with your teeth?

Does your water contain fluoride?

For Women Planning to Breastfeed

Do you have any questions about breastfeeding?

Have you attended any classes on breastfeeding?

Do you have family members or friends who will help as you are learning to breastfeed?

Do you know how to contact breastfeeding support groups or lactation consultants?

Do you know your HIV status?

For Parents Planning to Formula-Feed

Do you know what infant formula you plan to use? Is the infant formula iron fortified?

How will you prepare the infant formula?

After the infant formula is made, how will you store it?

Do you have family members or friends who will help you feed your baby?

Nutrition Counseling

For Pregnant Women

■ To minimize the risk of women giving birth to an infant with a neural tube defect, encourage them to consume folic acid, particularly before pregnancy and during the first trimester. Before pregnancy, women should consume 400 µg per day of folic acid (the synthetic form of folate) from fortified foods and/or supplements in addition to consuming a variety of foods that contain folate. Once pregnancy is confirmed, recommended intake is 600 dietary folate equivalents (DFEs) per day of food folate, folic acid, or a mixture of both.[10]

DFEs account for differences in the absorption of food folate and folic acid (i.e., 1 DFE equals 1 µg food folate, 0.6 µg folic acid [from fortified foods or supplements] consumed with food, or 0.5 µg folic acid [from supplements] taken on an empty stomach). Thus, 600 DFEs equal 600 µg food folate, 360 µg folic acid consumed with food, or 300 µg folic acid taken on an empty stomach.[10]

■ Inform women that concentrated sources of food folate include fruits (e.g., oranges, strawberries, avocados); dark-green leafy vegetables (e.g., spinach, turnip greens); some other vegetables (e.g., asparagus, broccoli, Brussels sprouts); and legumes (e.g., black, pinto, navy, and kidney beans). Folic acid can be obtained from fortified food products (e.g., fortified grain products, most ready-to-eat breakfast cereals).

■ Women should try to maintain a healthy weight throughout pregnancy.

■ Explain that a safe amount of alcohol consumption by pregnant women is not known. Therefore, the only sure way to avoid the possible harmful effects of alcohol on the fetus is to avoid drinking alcoholic beverages entirely.[9]

■ Encourage women who smoke to quit or cut back to improve their health and reduce the risk of giving birth to an infant with fetal growth retardation.[8]

■ Encourage women to maintain good oral hygiene and obtain dental care if needed.

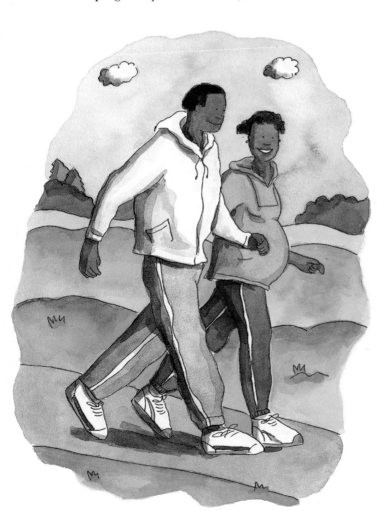

- Explain that weight loss after pregnancy should occur gradually by adjusting caloric intake, level of physical activity, or both.[9]

- Moderate physical activity, such as gentle aerobics (e.g., walking, swimming), is recommended as soon as possible after delivery to increase the mother's energy level.

For Women Planning to Breastfeed

- Encourage women to learn their HIV status. If they are HIV positive, breastfeeding is contra-indicated.

- Encourage women to try to keep their newborns in their rooms after delivery.

- Encourage women to begin breastfeeding their newborns as soon as possible after birth, usually within the first hour.[4]

- Instruct women to breastfeed when their newborns show signs of hunger (e.g., increased alertness or activity, mouthing, rooting). Tell women not to wait until their infants are crying; crying is the last indicator of hunger.[4]

- Instruct mothers to breastfeed their newborns approximately 8 to 12 times every 24 hours until they seem satisfied.[4]

- No supplements (e.g., water, glucose, formula) should be given to breastfeeding infants unless a medical condition requires it.[4]

For Parents Planning to Formula-Feed

- Instruct parents to prepare 2 oz of infant formula every 2 to 3 hours at first. More should be prepared if the infant seems hungry, especially as the infant grows.

- To reduce the infant's risk of developing early childhood caries, encourage parents to avoid doing things that may harm the infant's teeth (e.g., putting her to bed with a bottle, propping a bottle in her mouth, giving her a bottle when she's not hungry).

NEWBORN

Health professionals can use the general information in the section Nutrition Supervision Throughout Infancy (pp. 30–35), as well as the age-specific information that follows.

Interview Questions

For Parents of All Infants

What is the longest time Amanda has slept at one time?

How much rest are you getting?

How many wet diapers does Amanda have each day?

Do you burp her during or after a feeding?

Is anyone helping you feed Amanda?

For Mothers of Breastfed Infants

Do you have any questions about breastfeeding?

Do you need any help with breastfeeding?

How often do you feed Edward? How do you know when he is hungry?

Does Edward attach to your breast and suck well? Do you hear him make swallowing sounds when you breastfeed?

Have you had any problems with your breasts or nipples (for example, tenderness, swelling, or pain)?

Do you restrict any foods in your diet?

What vitamin or mineral supplements do you take or plan to take?

Do you drink wine, beer, or other alcoholic beverages?

Do you use any drugs (for example, prescription, over-the-counter, or illegal)?

Do you know your HIV status?

For Parents of Formula-Fed Infants

What infant formula do you use? Is the formula iron fortified?

How do you prepare the infant formula?

How do you store the infant formula after you make it?

How do you clean the nipples, bottles, and other equipment before and after feeding?

What do you do with the milk in the bottle after Amanda has finished eating?

How do you hold Amanda when you feed her?

Screening and Assessment

■ Perform metabolic screening as indicated by the state.

■ If the mother does not know her HIV status, suggest HIV screening.

■ If possible, observe the mother breastfeeding her infant. Assess the mother's comfort in feeding the infant, eye contact between the mother and infant, the mother's interaction with the infant, the mother's and infant's responses to distractions in the environment, and the infant's ability to suck. Help the mother and infant develop successful breastfeeding behaviors.

Nutrition Counseling

■ Instruct parents to feed the infant when she is hungry, typically 8 to 12 times in 24 hours. Signs of hunger include hand-to-mouth activity, rooting, pre-cry facial grimaces, fussing sounds, and crying.

■ Emphasize that the infant should be awakened for feeding during the first 2 weeks if the infant sleeps more than 4 hours at a time.[4]

■ Instruct parents to feed the infant until he seems full. Signs of fullness are turning his head away from the nipple, showing interest in things other than eating, and closing his mouth.

■ Encourage parents to burp the infant at natural breaks (e.g., midway through or after a feeding) by gently rubbing or patting her back while holding her against the shoulder and chest or supporting her in a sitting position on the lap.

■ Reassure parents that infants are getting enough milk if

They make swallowing sounds.

They have one or two wet and/or soiled diapers on the first day, increasing to six to eight wet cloth diapers or five or six disposable diapers and three or four stools every 24 hours. (The urine should be pale yellow, and stools should have the consistency of cottage cheese and be mustard-colored by the fourth day.)

They are gaining weight appropriately.

■ Encourage mothers to breastfeed the infant exclusively for the first 6 months. Explain that breastfeeding provides ideal nutrition and promotes the best possible growth and development.

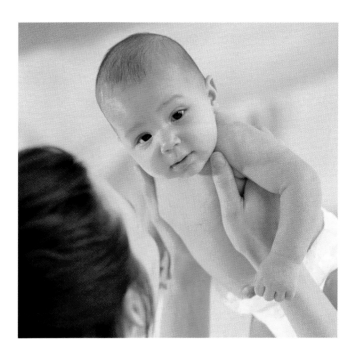

Water, juice, and other foods are generally unnecessary for breastfed infants.[4]

■ Explain to parents that neither breastfed nor formula-fed infants need to drink fluoridated water or take fluoride supplements during the first 6 months.[4]

Are you planning to return to work or school? If so, are you expressing your breastmilk? How do you store it? How long do you keep it?

For Parents of Formula-Fed Infants

What infant formula are you feeding Carmen? Is it iron fortified?

How often do you feed her? How much does she eat at a feeding?

Have you offered Carmen anything other than infant formula?

What do you do with infant formula left in the bottle when she has finished eating?

Do you have any concerns about the infant formula (for example, cost, preparation, amount, or nutrient content)?

Screening and Assessment

■ Assess the need for vitamin D or iron supplementation.

Nutrition Counseling

■ Emphasize to parents that infants should not be offered food other than breastmilk or infant formula until they can sit with support and have good control of the head and neck, at about 4 to 6 months. At this time, infants may be ready to try an iron-fortified, single-grain infant cereal (e.g., rice cereal).

■ Explain that no nutritional advantage is known, but disadvantages may exist, in introducing supplemental foods before the infant is developmentally ready, at about 4 to 6 months.[6]

■ Encourage parents to gradually offer fruits and vegetables after the infant has accepted iron-fortified, single-grain infant cereal.

■ Emphasize that before 6 months of age, infants should not be fed spinach, beets, turnips, carrots, or collard greens canned at home or by the manufacturer because they may contain too much nitrate, which can cause methemoglobinemia (also called blue baby syndrome).[6]

■ Instruct parents to offer new foods one at a time and to observe their infants for 7 days or more after a new food is introduced to make sure they do not have an adverse reaction (e.g., a rash).

■ Explain that after infants eat several types of fruits and vegetables, they can try well-cooked, strained or pureed meats with iron (e.g., lean beef, pork, chicken, turkey).

■ Reassure parents that it is normal for infants to drool more at 3 to 4 months of age as their salivary glands become more active.

■ Explain to parents that neither breastfed nor formula-fed infants need to drink fluoridated water or take fluoride supplements during the first 6 months.[4]

■ Inform parents that infant toys encourage physical activity. Playing with safe, age-appropriate toys (e.g., rattles, stuffed animals, plastic toys) and moving them from hand to mouth and sucking and gumming them helps infants develop skills they will use later when they feed themselves.

■ Encourage parents to talk to the infant during feedings. As infants develop, they increasingly respond to social interaction.

6 MONTHS

Health professionals can use the general information in the section Nutrition Supervision Throughout Infancy (pp. 30–35), as well as the age-specific information that follows.

Interview Questions

For Parents of All Infants

Can Rebecca wait without crying while you get ready to feed her?

When does Rebecca have something to eat or drink? How much does she eat or drink at a time? What does she do when she has had enough to eat?

How does Rebecca let you know when she likes a certain food? Does she have favorite foods? If so, what are they?

Has she eaten any foods from the family meal? If so, which ones?

Has Rebecca fed herself anything?

Has she put any nonfood items in her mouth? If so, what were they? Did she swallow them?

Do you know what Rebecca is fed when she is away from home (for example, at child care)?

Has Rebecca's first tooth erupted? Has she had any teething problems?

For Mothers of Breastfed Infants

Do you have any questions about breastfeeding?

How often does Paul breastfeed? How long do you feed him each time?

Has he received breastmilk or other fluids from a bottle or cup?

Have you given Paul any infant formula or cow's, goat's, or soy milk?

For Parents of Formula-Fed Infants

How often do you feed Rebecca? How much infant formula does she drink at a time?

Have you offered her anything other than infant formula?

Does Rebecca want to help hold her bottle?

Do you have any concerns about the infant formula (for example, cost, preparation, amount, or nutrient content)?

What kind of water is used to prepare the formula? Does the water contain fluoride?

Screening and Assessment

■ Assess the need for vitamin D or iron supplementation.

■ Assess all sources of water used by the family (including municipal, well, commercially bottled, and home system–processed) and ready-to-feed infant formula manufactured without fluoridated water to determine the need for fluoride supplementation. If the infant is not getting enough fluoride, refer the infant to a physician or dentist.

Nutrition Counseling

■ Instruct parents to feed the infant when he is hungry. Signs of hunger include hand-to-mouth activity, rooting, pre-cry facial grimaces, fussing sounds, and crying.

- Instruct parents to introduce supplemental foods to the infant when her sucking reflex has changed to allow coordinated swallowing, she can sit with support, and she has good head and neck control.

- Instruct parents to use a spoon when offering the infant a new food and to place the infant in a sitting position.

- Emphasize that if the infant does not like a new food, she should not be forced to eat it. The food can be offered at a later time. It may take 15 to 20 attempts before an infant accepts a particular food.

- Instruct parents to offer new foods one at a time and to observe their infants for 7 days or more after a new food is introduced to make sure they do not have an adverse reaction (e.g., a rash).

- Instruct parents to offer the infant a wide variety of foods.

- Explain that infants receiving infant formula not fortified with iron need two or more servings per day of iron-fortified infant cereal to meet their iron requirements.[5]

- Tell parents to offer the infant fruits and vegetables after he has accepted iron-fortified infant cereal. One feeding per day of fruits and/or vegetables rich in vitamin C helps the infant absorb iron.[5]

- Inform parents that after the infant eats several types of fruits and vegetables, she can try well-cooked, strained or pureed meats with iron (e.g., lean beef, pork, chicken, turkey).

- Encourage parents to offer the infant finger foods (e.g., green beans, cereal, crackers) when he can eat solid foods.

- Inform parents that they can offer store-bought and home-prepared baby food, but infants who can feed themselves soft foods do not need it.

- Tell parents that infants do not need salt, spices, or sugar added to their food.

- Explain that a highchair allows the infant to be part of the family circle at mealtime, but a safety belt should be used to secure her.

- Instruct parents to clean the infant's gums and teeth twice a day. A clean, moist washcloth can be used to wipe the gums. A small, soft toothbrush (without toothpaste) and water can be used to clean the teeth.

- Inform parents that by 6 months of age, infants become very active and benefit from playing with toys for stacking, shaking, pushing, or dropping and from playing with others. Encourage parents to include the infant in family play times.

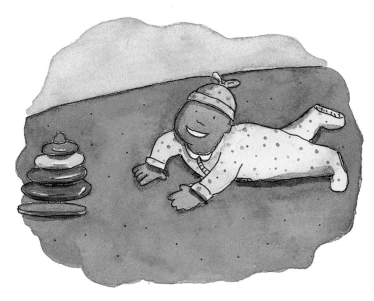

9 MONTHS

Health professionals can use the general information in the section Nutrition Supervision Throughout Infancy (pp. 30–35), as well as the age-specific information that follows.

Interview Questions

For Parents of All Infants

Who feeds Bonnie?

When does Bonnie have something to eat or drink? How much does she eat or drink at a time? What does she do when she has had enough to eat?

Is Bonnie interested in feeding herself?

What foods does Bonnie eat with her fingers? Has she used a cup?

Is Bonnie interested in the food you eat?

Do you know what Bonnie eats when she is away from home (for example, at child care)?

Is Bonnie drinking less breastmilk or infant formula?

Has she ever choked or gagged on food?

Has Bonnie's first tooth erupted? Does she have any teething problems?

For Mothers of Breastfed Infants

How often does Juan breastfeed? How long do you feed him each time?

How is your milk supply?

Has Juan had infant formula or cow's, goat's, or soy milk?

For Parents of Formula-Fed Infants

How much infant formula does Bonnie drink?

Are you using fluoridated water to prepare her infant formula?

Do you have any questions about weaning Bonnie from the bottle?

Screening and Assessment

■ Screen the infant for iron-deficiency anemia if any of these risk factors are present (see the Iron-Deficiency Anemia chapter):[5]

Was born preterm or with low birthweight

Was fed non–iron-fortified infant formula for more than 2 months

Was fed cow's milk before 12 months

Consumes more than 24 oz of cow's milk daily

Is breastfed and doesn't get enough iron

Is from a family with low income

Is eligible for WIC

Is from a migrant family

Is from a family of recently arrived refugees

Has special health care needs (e.g., takes medications that interfere with iron absorption; has chronic infection, inflammatory disorders, restricted diets, extensive blood loss from a wound, an accident, or surgery)

- Screen the infant for lead exposure. (See Appendix E: Screening for Elevated Blood Lead Levels.)

- Assess the need for neurological evaluation if the infant stiffens during feeding, retains oral reflexes such as rooting, experiences delays in learning feeding skills, or refuses textured food when developmentally ready (i.e., textural aversion).

- Assess all sources of water used by the family (including municipal, well, commercially bottled, and home system–processed) and ready-to-feed infant formula manufactured without fluoridated water to determine the need for fluoride supplementation. If the infant is not getting enough fluoride, refer the infant to a physician or dentist.

Nutrition Counseling

- Instruct parents to offer soft, moist foods (e.g., mashed potatoes and other cooked vegetables, spaghetti with sauce, rice, tuna, meat loaf) as the infant gradually changes from gumming to chewing foods.

- Explain that as the infant gains more control over picking up and holding food, small pieces of soft foods can be offered.

- Encourage parents to be patient and understanding as the infant tries new foods and learns to feed herself.

- Encourage parents to remove distractions so that the infant stays focused on the food.

- Explain that a highchair allows the infant to be part of the family circle at mealtime, but a safety belt should be used to secure him.

- Instruct parents to clean the infant's gums and teeth twice a day. A clean, moist washcloth can be used to wipe the gums. A small, soft toothbrush (without toothpaste) and water can be used to clean the teeth.

- Infants should be encouraged to drink from a cup with assistance.

- Most 9-month-olds are on the same eating schedule as the family: breakfast, lunch, and dinner. Instruct parents to give the infant snacks midmorning, in the afternoon, and at bedtime.

- If infants are fed away from home, parents need to know what and how much they eat.

- Most infants are crawling by 9 months and may begin to walk by holding onto furniture. Warn parents never to put the infant in a walker because of the risk of severe injury or death. Parents can physically support the infant as she plays and explores her newly found strength and agility.

Table 1. Desired Outcomes for the Infant, and the Role of the Family

Infant

Educational/Attitudinal	Behavioral	Health
■ Has a sense of trust ■ Bonds with parents ■ Enjoys eating	■ Breastfeeds successfully ■ Bottle feeds successfully if not breastfeeding ■ Consumes supplemental foods to support appropriate growth and development	■ Develops normal rooting, sucking, and swallowing reflexes ■ Develops fine and gross motor skills ■ Grows and develops at an appropriate rate ■ Maintains good health

Family

Educational/Attitudinal	Behavioral	Health
■ Bonds with the infant ■ Enjoys feeding the infant ■ Understands the infant's nutrition needs ■ Acquires a sense of competence in meeting the infant's needs ■ Understands the importance of a healthy lifestyle, including healthy eating behaviors and regular physical activity, to promote short-term and long-term health	■ Meets the infant's nutrition needs ■ Responds to infant's hunger and satiety cues ■ Holds the infant when breastfeeding or bottle feeding and maintains eye contact ■ Talks to the infant during feeding ■ Provides a pleasant eating environment ■ Uses nutrition programs and food resources if needed ■ Seeks help when problems occur	■ Maintains good health

References

1. Trahms CM, Pipes PL. 1997. *Nutrition in Infancy and Childhood* (6th ed.). New York, NY: WCB/McGraw-Hill.

2. American Dental Association. 1998. *ADA Guide to Dental Therapeutics*. Chicago, IL: ADA Publishing.

3. World Health Organization, Division of Child Health and Development. 1998. *Evidence for the Ten Steps to Successful Breastfeeding*. Geneva, Switzerland: World Health Organization, Division of Child Health and Development.

4. American Academy of Pediatrics, Work Group on Breastfeeding. 1997. Breastfeeding and the use of human milk. *Pediatrics* 100(6):1035–1039.

5. Centers for Disease Control and Prevention, Epidemiology Program Office. 1998. *Recommendations to Prevent and Control Iron Deficiency in the United States*. Atlanta, GA: Centers for Disease Control and Prevention, Epidemiology Program Office.

6. Kleinman RE, ed. 1999. *Pediatric Nutrition Handbook* (4th ed.). Elk Grove Village, IL: American Academy of Pediatrics.

7. Graves DE, Suitor CW, Holt KA, eds. 1997. *Making Food Healthy and Safe for Children: How to Meet the National Health and Safety Performance Standards—Guidelines for Out-of-Home Child Care Programs*. Arlington, VA: National Center for Education in Maternal and Child Health.

8. Dietz WH, Stern L, eds. 1999. *Guide to Your Child's Nutrition: Making Peace at the Table and Building Healthy Eating Habits for Life*. New York, NY: Villard Books.

9. National Academy of Sciences, Institute of Medicine, Food and Nutrition Board. 1992. *Nutrition During Pregnancy and Lactation: An Implementation Guide*. Washington, DC: National Academy Press.

10. National Academy of Sciences, Institute of Medicine, Food and Nutrition Board. 1998. *Dietary Reference Intakes for Thiamin, Riboflavin, Niacin, Vitamin B_6, Folate, Vitamin B_{12}, Pantothenic Acid, Biotin, and Choline*. Washington, DC: National Academy Press.

Suggested Reading

Fitzsimons D, Dwyer JT, Palmer C, Boyd L. 1998. Nutrition and oral health guidelines for pregnant women, infants, and children. *Journal of The American Dietetic Association* 98(2):182–189.

Fomon S, ed. 1993. *Nutrition of Normal Infants*. St. Louis, MO: Mosby-Year Book.

Green M, Palfrey JS, eds. 2000. *Bright Futures: Guidelines for Health Supervision of Infants, Children, and Adolescents* (2nd ed.). Arlington, VA: National Center for Education in Maternal and Child Health.

Tsang TC, Zlotkin SH, Nichols BL, Hansen JW. 1997. *Nutrition During Infancy: Principles and Practice* (2nd ed.). Cincinnati, OH: Digital Educational Publishers.

Walker WA, Watkins JB. 1997. *Nutrition in Pediatrics*. Hamilton, Ontario, Canada: BC Decker.

Worthington-Roberts BS, Williams SR. 1997. *Nutrition in Pregnancy and Lactation* (6th ed.). Madison, WI: Brown and Benchmark Publishers.

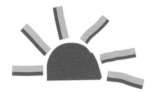

Successfully Introducing Solid Foods

John's mother is careful to offer new foods one at a time and to observe John for 7 days or more to make sure he does not have an adverse reaction.

John Matthews is a 5-month-old infant who has been fed only breastmilk. He is 27 inches long and weighs 18 pounds. Both his length and weight have been between the 75th and 90th percentiles since he was 2 months old. Lately, his appetite appears to have increased.

At the health clinic, John's mother tells Liz Roberts, the dietitian, that her son seems to want to breastfeed all the time, and she wonders whether it would be all right to add some solid foods to his diet. The dietitian confirmed that John has good head and neck control and can maintain a sitting position with little or no assistance. His sucking pattern has changed from the weaker, up-and-down movements of early infancy to stronger, back-and-forth movements. He is able to grasp objects that are placed within his reach, and he brings them to his mouth. He no longer exhibits the "tongue thrust" motion when a spoon or object is placed in his mouth.

Ms. Roberts advises mixing a small amount of iron-fortified rice cereal with expressed breastmilk and offering it to John on a spoon. She recommends that John's mother try feeding him the cereal when he is well rested and slightly hungry.

When John's mother first feeds him the rice cereal, he looks surprised but swallows it. He accepts a second spoonful, then turns his head away. The next day, John's mother offers him the cereal mixture again, and he eagerly eats four spoonfuls. She slowly increases the amount of cereal to several tablespoons.

Over the next few weeks, John's mother gradually begins to introduce fruits and vegetables into John's diet. She is careful to offer new foods one at a time and to observe John for 7 days or more to make sure he does not have an adverse reaction. John continues to breastfeed on demand.

FREQUENTLY ASKED QUESTIONS
ABOUT NUTRITION IN INFANCY

■ Should I breastfeed or use infant formula?

Breastmilk is the ideal food for babies.

Even if you breastfeed for only a few weeks or months, there are many benefits for you and your baby. Breastfeeding helps your baby resist colds, ear infections, allergies, and other illnesses.

If for any reason you feel you cannot breastfeed (for example, you have to work or go to school, or you are worried about not producing enough breastmilk), talk to a health professional, breastfeeding specialist, or breastfeeding support group. They can answer questions and help you come up with solutions. Your family and friends are also sources of support.

If your baby has special health care needs, you may still be able to breastfeed. You may need help with positioning, special equipment, and additional support from family and friends.

If you decide to use infant formula, your health professional can help you choose the right type of formula and answer your questions about feeding.

■ How do I know if my baby is getting enough breastmilk?

Your baby may show she is hungry by sucking, putting her hands to her mouth, opening and closing her mouth, or looking for the nipple. She shows she is full by falling asleep after breastfeeding.

As a general rule, your baby will have five to eight wet diapers and three or four stools a day by the time she's 5 to 7 days old.

Your baby will be gaining weight. (A full-term baby should be back to her birthweight by 10 days to 2 weeks of age. After that she should gain 5 to 7 oz a week and should double her birthweight by 4 to 6 months of age.)

■ What is colic? How can I prevent or manage it?

When your baby cries without apparent reason for several hours on a regular basis, he may have colic. Colic occurs in almost 10 percent of babies. No one knows what causes colic—it is not caused by poor parenting. Colic usually develops between 2 and 6 weeks of age and disappears by 3 or 4 months.

There is no cure for colic. Here are some tips to help manage colic as you wait for your baby to outgrow it:

- If you are breastfeeding, try avoiding some foods, such as cow's milk, wheat, peanuts, eggs, and seafood.

- Cuddle and rock your baby during crying bouts.

- Swaddle your baby or apply firm but gentle pressure to the stomach.

- Darken the room or play soft music.

- Get help so you can take time off from caring for your baby.

■ When and how should I introduce solid foods?

Introduce solid foods when your baby is ready, at about 4 to 6 months of age. Each baby is different, so you need to learn your baby's cues. Can he sit up by himself for a while? Does he have good control of his head and neck? Can he pick up food with his fist?

Offer rice cereal as the first solid food, because it is least likely to cause an allergic reaction.

Do not add cereal to bottles, and do not use "baby food nurser kits."

Solid foods are usually introduced in this order: iron-fortified infant cereal, then fruits, vegetables, and meats. After you introduce cereal, you can introduce the rest in any order you wish.

Offer foods your baby is able to eat.

Introduce one food at a time, waiting 7 days or more to see how your baby tolerates the food.

Introduce foods that are more likely to cause an allergic reaction (for example, citrus fruits, berries, and wheat) last.

Puree foods prepared for the family meal and serve them to your baby.

Do not add sugar or salt to your baby's food.

Most store-bought foods provide adequate nutrition, but check the labels to make sure they have no additives, sugar, or salt.

By 1 year of age, your baby should be eating a wide range of foods.

■ **When should I introduce juice and how much?**

When your baby seems ready, at 4 to 6 months or later, introduce juice by using a cup.

Give your baby juice in a cup, not a bottle, because juice in a bottle can bathe her teeth in sugar for long periods of time. Juice in a bottle also makes it harder to wean your baby from a bottle.

Although juices provide carbohydrates and vitamin C, do not use them instead of breastmilk or infant formula.

Offer juice in small amounts. A reasonable amount of juice is 4 oz per day. Too much juice (more than 8 to 10 oz per day) may decrease your baby's appetite for other foods and increase the risk of loose stools and diarrhea.

■ **How can I protect my baby's teeth from tooth decay?**

To prevent early childhood caries (baby bottle tooth decay), do not allow your baby to suck on a bottle of juice, sweetened drinks, or milk for long periods of time. Signs of caries include white spots on the teeth near the gums.

Do not put your baby to bed with a bottle or allow him to have a bottle whenever he wants.

Clean the infant's gums and teeth twice a day. A clean, moist washcloth can be used to wipe the gums. A small, soft toothbrush (without toothpaste) and water can be used to clean the teeth.

■ **How can I tell if my baby is ready to feed herself?**

If your baby can pick up food and chew or mash it, she is ready to feed herself soft pieces of table food.

■ **When should I wean my baby from the bottle?**

As your baby begins to eat more solid foods and drink from a cup, he can be weaned from the bottle. Wean your baby gradually, at about 9 to 10 months. By 12 to 14 months, most babies are drinking from a cup.

■ When should I give my baby cow's milk?

You may give your baby cow's milk, goat's milk, or soy milk after her first birthday.

Do not give your baby low-fat or nonfat milk. She needs the extra fat in whole milk for growth and development.

■ Should I give my baby sweets?

Do not give your baby sweets (for example, candy, cake, or cookies). He needs to eat healthy foods for growth and development.

After the first year, your child can have sweets in moderation.

■ Many members of my family are overweight. How can I prevent my baby from becoming overweight?

Breastfeed if possible.

Learn your baby's hunger cues and feed her when she's hungry. Feeding to calm her or to relieve boredom teaches her to use food as a source of comfort.

Teach your baby to use other means for comfort (for example, cuddling, rocking, talking, and walking).

Feed your baby until she is full. Don't force her to finish a bottle or other food.

Don't add cereal to the bottle—this may cause your baby to eat more than she needs. She may also choke on the cereal.

Feed your baby slowly. Don't enlarge the hole in the bottle nipple to make the milk come out faster. It takes about 20 minutes for your baby to feel full.

Do not give your baby sweets during the first 12 months.

■ What can I expect my baby to do as he grows?

Newborn to 1 Month

Your baby will have rooting, sucking, and swallowing reflexes.

He will begin to develop the ability to start and stop sucking.

He will wake up and fall asleep easily.

3 to 4 Months

Your baby will smile.

She will raise her head when she is on her stomach.

She will drool more.

She will follow objects and sounds with her eyes.

She will put her hand in her mouth a lot.

She will sit with support.

6 Months

Your baby will begin to eat solid foods at about 4 to 6 months.

He will smile responsively and babble.

His torso will move in the direction of his neck when he turns his head while lying on his back.

He will reach for objects and pick them up with one hand.

He will hold his hands together.

He will sit with support.

7 to 9 Months

Your baby will try to grasp foods (for example, melba toast, crackers, and teething biscuits) with her palms. She will not be able to pick them up with her fingers.

9 to 12 Months

Your baby will pinch food with his fingers and try to feed himself.

He will try to use a cup.

He may be shy and anxious around strangers.

He will respond to his name and familiar people.

He will play games such as peek-a-boo.

He will make a variety of sounds, and by 1 year he may speak several words.

He will explore toys with his eyes and mouth, and will transfer a toy from one hand to the other.

He will sit and crawl, and may walk without support.

Resources for Health Professionals and Families

Dietz WH, Stern L, eds. 1999. *Guide to Your Child's Nutrition: Making Peace at the Table and Building Healthy Eating Habits for Life*. New York, NY: Villard Books.

Dunn AM, Evers C. 1996. Nutrition. In Burns CE, Barber N, Brady AM, Dunn AM. *Pediatric Primary Care: A Handbook for Nurse Practitioners*. Philadelphia, PA: WB Saunders.

Schmidt BDC. 1992. *Instructions for Pediatric Patients*. Philadelphia, PA: WB Saunders.

Trahms CM, Pipes PL. 1997. *Nutrition in Infancy and Childhood* (6th ed.). New York, NY: WCB/McGraw-Hill.

Worthington-Roberts BS, Williams SR. 1997. *Nutrition in Pregnancy and Lactation* (6th ed.). Madison, WI: Brown and Benchmark Publishers.

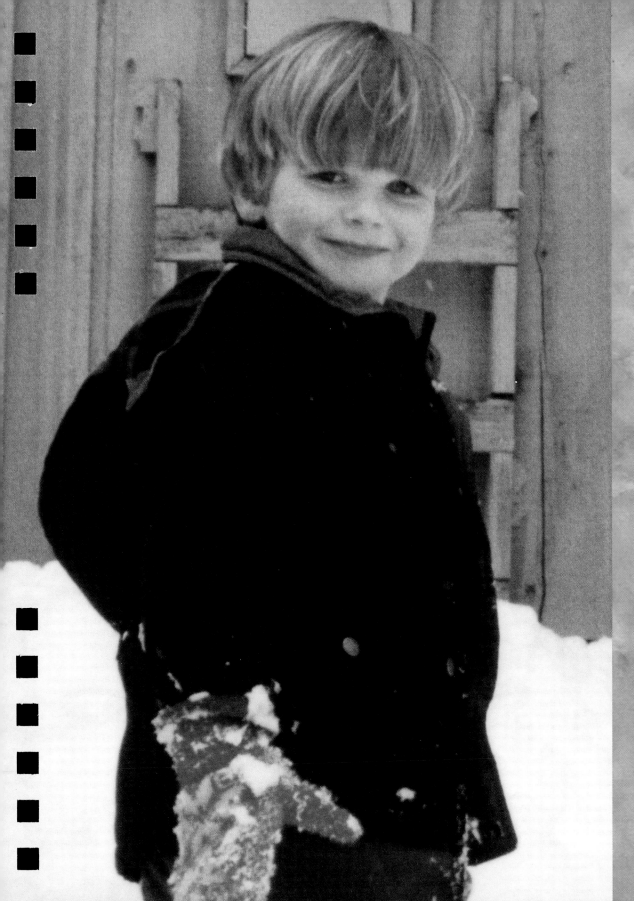

Early Childhood

1–4 Years

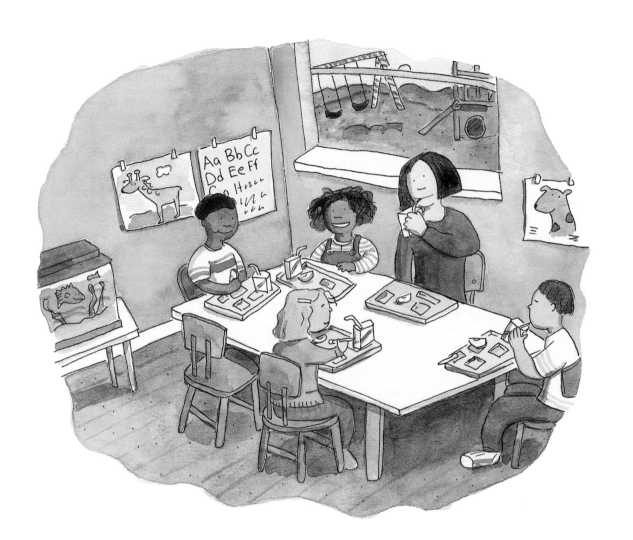

EARLY CHILDHOOD

During early childhood, a child's world expands to include friends, school-mates, and others in the community. The child's physical, cognitive, social, and emotional development are tightly linked. For example, nutrition affects not only the physical health of children but also their emotional health. When offered developmentally appropriate food in a supportive environment, children can thrive.

Early childhood is divided into two stages: the toddler stage, ages 1 to 2, and the young child stage, ages 3 to 4. The toddler stage can be stressful for parents as toddlers develop a sense of independence. In addition, toddlers may struggle with their parents over food. By 3 years old, young children usually are more competent at feeding themselves. As they get older, young children become more interested in trying new foods, and they enjoy participating in family meals.

Practicing healthy eating behaviors during early childhood is essential for

- Promoting optimal growth, development, and health.

- Preventing immediate health problems (e.g., iron-deficiency anemia, undernutrition, obesity, early childhood caries).

- Laying the foundation for lifelong health and reducing the risk of chronic disease (e.g., cardio-vascular disease, type 2 diabetes mellitus, hypertension, some forms of cancer, osteoporosis).

Growth and Physical Development

A child's birthweight quadruples by 2 years of age. Between the ages of 2 and 5, children gain an average of 4.5 to 6.5 pounds per year and grow 2.5 to 3.5 inches per year. As the growth rate declines during early childhood, a child's appetite decreases and the amount of food consumed may become unpredictable.[1]

During early childhood, children predominantly use their cheeks rather than their tongues to swallow. As toddlers' eating skills develop, they progress from eating soft pieces of food to foods with more texture. By age 3 or 4, they are able to

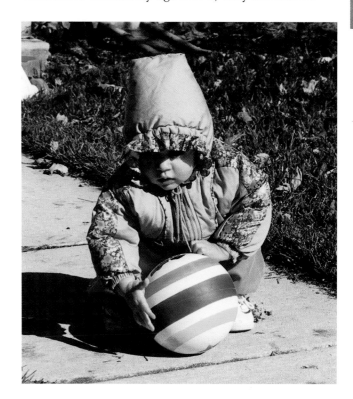

use their fingers to push food on a spoon, pick up food with a fork, and drink from a cup. Children do not have the muscle control yet to cut their food or eat all foods neatly.

Children who are bottle fed should be weaned from the bottle and encouraged to use a cup at about 12 to 14 months of age. The risk for early childhood caries (baby bottle tooth decay) increases if children are allowed to suck on a bottle filled with any liquid except water for prolonged periods.

Social and Emotional Development

The Toddler: 1 to 2 Years

Toddlers tend to be leery of new foods and may refuse to eat them. They need to look at the new foods and touch, smell, feel, and taste them—perhaps as many as 15 to 20 times before they accept them.[2,3]

Toddlers are unpredictable. The foods they like one day may be different the next. They may eat a lot one day, and very little the next. Unlike adults, they usually eat only one or two foods at a meal. Parents often become alarmed when toddlers' eating behaviors change so much, and often so abruptly.

Parents should not become concerned that their toddler is not eating enough. Toddlers' growth rates decrease during early childhood; therefore, their energy needs decrease. Despite these changes, toddlers will consume a variety of foods if parents continue to serve developmentally appropriate healthy meals and snacks.

To encourage toddlers to establish healthy eating behaviors, parents need to provide a structured,

but pleasant, mealtime environment and serve as role models by eating a variety of foods. Parents are responsible for what, when, and where the toddler eats; toddlers are responsible for whether to eat and how much.[3]

The Young Child: 3 to 4 Years

Around age 3 or 4, young children become more curious about food, although they still may be reluctant to try new foods. This reluctance can be overcome if parents talk about new foods and allow their children to prepare and perhaps grow them.

As young children grow, they become less impulsive and can follow instructions. They can stay calm when they are hungry, join in conversation during mealtimes, serve themselves, and pass food to others. Young children are more comfortable eating in unfamiliar places than they were as toddlers.

Young children should be encouraged to try new foods. The goal is for children to accept a variety of healthy foods—not simply to get them to eat what is on their plates.

Healthy Lifestyles

Early childhood is a key time for promoting the development of motor skills and good habits for physical activity that will last a lifetime. Most children are active but may not have the opportunity to play and explore because of space or safety concerns.

Physical activities (e.g., running, jumping, climbing; throwing, catching, or hitting a ball) should be encouraged. Simple games such as "Simon says," chase, and tag are appropriate during early childhood. Organized activities tailored to the developmental needs of children (e.g., gymnastics, swimming, dancing) are also appropriate. Because most children need to develop their motor skills, they are not ready for organized, competitive sports, which require visual acuity, control, and balance.

Partnerships with the Community

Partnerships among health professionals, families, and communities are essential for ensuring that parents receive guidance on childhood nutrition and feeding. Health professionals give parents the opportunity to discuss nutrition issues and concerns affecting their children and can identify and contact community resources to help parents feed their children.

Many children spend time with child care providers or participate in Head Start or other preschool programs, which provide opportunities for promoting healthy eating behaviors. Children in community programs can be introduced to new foods and may try them more readily if their peers seem to be enjoying them.

By directly providing food and vouchers for food, nutrition programs ensure that families with low incomes have access to food.

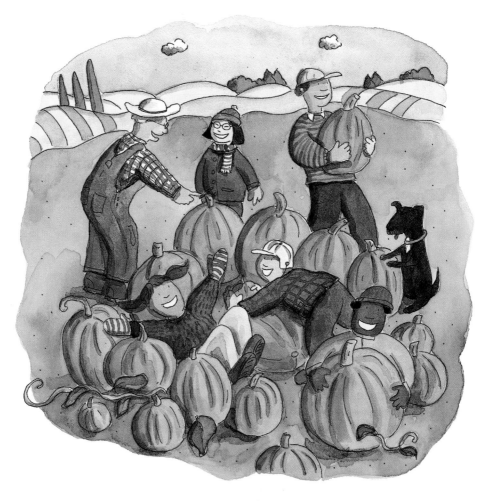

Federally funded food assistance and nutrition programs can provide a substantial part of a child's daily nutrition requirements. (See Appendix K: Federal Food Assistance and Nutrition Programs.) Food shelves and pantries, churches and other places of worship, and businesses can also provide food.

Common Nutrition Concerns

The most important nutrition message for parents during early childhood is to ensure that their children consume enough calories and nutrients to support adequate growth and development. Before children are 2, their fat intake should not be restricted. After 2 years of age, children should gradually eat fewer high-fat foods, so that by 5 years of age they are getting no more than 30 percent of their daily calories from fat (33 g per 1,000 kcal).[2] As they begin to consume fewer calories from fat, children should eat more grain products, fruits and vegetables, low-fat dairy products, lean meats, and other protein-rich foods.

Iron-deficiency anemia may have adverse effects on growth and development. Iron-deficiency anemia is common in children and is especially prevalent among children from families with low incomes. The prevalence of iron-deficiency anemia can be reduced by doing the following:[4]

- Waiting until children are 12 months of age before feeding them cow's milk

- Offering children no more than 16 oz of cow's milk daily

- Encouraging consumption of iron-rich foods (e.g., meat, fish, poultry) and foods that contain vitamin C (e.g., fruits, vegetables, juice), which enhances iron absorption

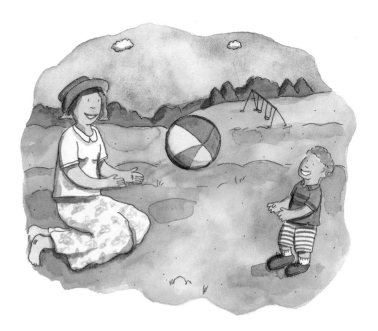

Children with special health care needs may have nutrition concerns, including poor growth, poor eating skills, inadequate food intake, developmental delays, elimination problems, and metabolic disorders. These children may need specialized care from a dietitian; they may also need referral to early intervention programs in their communities.

A child's nutrition status should be evaluated during comprehensive nutrition supervision visits or as part of general health supervision visits. (For more information on health supervision, see *Bright Futures: Guidelines for Health Supervision of Infants, Children, and Adolescents,* listed under Suggested Reading in this chapter.)

Health professionals begin nutrition supervision by gathering information about the child's nutrition status. This can be accomplished by selectively asking key interview questions listed in this chapter or by reviewing a questionnaire filled out by parents before the visit. (See Appendix B: Nutrition Questionnaire for Children.) These methods provide a useful starting point for identifying nutrition concerns.

Health professionals can then use this chapter's screening and assessment guidelines, and nutrition counseling guidelines, to provide families with anticipatory guidance. Nutrition supervision information that pertains to the entire early childhood developmental period (Nutrition Supervision Throughout Early Childhood) is provided first in this chapter, followed by information for age-specific visits. Interview questions, screening and assessment, and nutrition counseling should be used as appropriate and will vary from visit to visit and from child to child.

To assist health professionals in promoting optimal nutrition that will last a lifetime, desired outcomes for the child and responsibilities for the family are identified in Table 2.

Nutrition Supervision Throughout Early Childhood

Interview Questions

Do you have any concerns about Marla's eating behaviors or growth?

How does she let you know when she is hungry and when she is full?

What do you do if Marla doesn't like a particular food?

Do you enjoy sharing meals and snacks with her?

Do you have appropriate equipment for feeding Marla (for example, cups, eating utensils, and an infant seat, highchair, or booster seat)?

Do you have any concerns about the food served to her when she is away from home?

What is the source of your drinking and cooking water? Do you use bottled or processed water?

Are you concerned about having enough money to buy food?

Screening and Assessment

■ Measure the child's length or height and weight, and plot these on a standard growth chart (e.g., the revised Centers for Disease Control and Prevention [CDC]/National Center for Health Statistics [NCHS] growth chart). Deviation from the expected growth pattern (e.g., a major change in growth percentiles on the chart) should be evaluated. This may be normal or may indicate a nutrition problem (e.g., difficulties with eating).

63

- Length or height and weight measurements can be used to indicate nutrition and growth status. Changes in weight reflect a child's short-term nutrient intake and serve as general indicators of nutrition status and overall health. Low height-for-age reflects long-term, cumulative nutrition or health problems.

- Body mass index (BMI) can be used as a screening tool to determine nutrition status and overall health. Calculate the child's BMI by dividing weight by the square of height (kg/m^2) or by referring to a BMI chart. Compare the BMI to the norms listed for the child's sex and age on the chart.

- Evaluate the appearance of the child's skin, hair, teeth, gums, tongue, and eyes.

- Assess fluoride levels in all sources of water used by the family (including municipal, well, commercially bottled, and home system–processed) to determine the need for fluoride supplementation. If the child is not getting enough fluoride, refer the child to a physician or dentist.

- Assess eating behaviors to determine the child's risk for early childhood caries (baby bottle tooth decay).

- Ask whether the child has regular dental checkups.

- Evaluate the child's progress in developing eating skills (including chewing and swallowing).

Nutrition Counseling

Health professionals can use the following information to provide anticipatory guidance to parents. Anticipatory guidance provides information on the child's nutrition status and on what to expect as the child enters the next developmental period, and promotes a positive attitude about food and healthy eating behaviors. (For additional information on nutrition counseling, see Appendix G: Strategies for Health Professionals to Promote Healthy Eating Behaviors.)

Parent-Child Feeding Relationship

- Inform parents that they are responsible for what, when, and where the child eats. To ensure that the child's nutrition needs are met, parents need to

  Purchase and prepare food.

  Serve developmentally appropriate and healthy food at scheduled times.

  Make meal and snack times pleasant.

  Make sure the child develops eating skills (e.g., progresses from using her hands for eating to using utensils).[5]

- Children are responsible for deciding whether to eat and how much.[5]

Eating Behaviors

- Emphasize to parents that children need healthy meals and snacks at scheduled times throughout the day to help them achieve nutritional balance.[6]

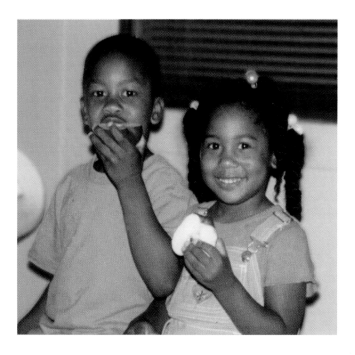

- Tell parents that children are unpredictable in the amounts and types of foods they eat, from meal to meal and from day to day. Reassure parents that children usually eat enough food to meet their nutrition needs.

- Instruct parents to modify foods to make them easier for the child to eat.

- From ages 2 to 5, children make the transition from the higher fat intake necessary in infancy to the lower fat intake recommended for the rest of the population. Inform parents that the children's fat intake should gradually be reduced to no more than 30 percent of their daily calories by age 5.[2]

- Tell parents that children 2 to 3 years of age need the same number of servings as children 4 to 6, but they may need smaller portions—about 2/3 of a serving.[6]

- Explain that by the time children are 4, they can eat serving sizes similar to those eaten by older family members (e.g., 1/2 cup of fruits or vegetables; 3/4 cup of juice; 1 slice of bread; 2 to 3 oz of cooked lean meat, poultry, or fish).

- Instruct parents to serve children 1 to 2 years of age whole milk. For older children, 2 percent, low-fat, or skim milk is acceptable.[2]

- Instruct parents to offer two servings of milk per day to children 2 to 6.[6] Excessive milk intake can reduce the child's appetite for other foods.

- Encourage parents to wean the child from the bottle by 12 to 14 months.

- Instruct parents to serve juice in a cup instead of a bottle and to limit the child's consumption of juice to 4 oz per day.

- Explain that children who drink fruit juices or sweetened beverages (e.g., Kool-Aid, fruit punch, soft drinks) whenever they want are at increased risk for early childhood caries and minor infections, and may experience loose stools and diarrhea.

- Emphasize that children who consume foods (e.g., candy, cookies) and beverages high in sugar (e.g., Kool-Aid, fruit punch) in unlimited amounts are likely to fill up on these foods rather than eat healthy foods.

- Encourage parents to make sure the child drinks plenty of water throughout the day.

Mealtimes

- Explain to parents that meals and snacks can be important social times for children. Parents should turn off the television and make mealtimes a pleasant experience.

65

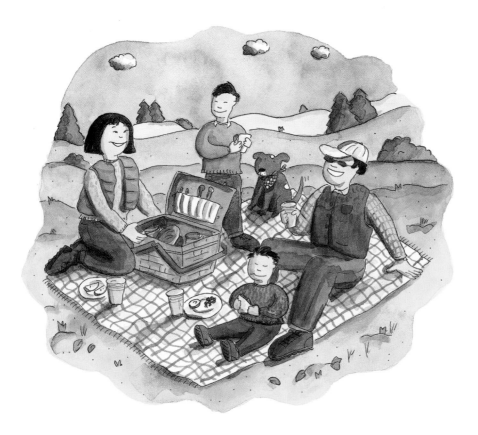

- Emphasize that children eat better when an adult is nearby, particularly when the adult shares the meal or snack with them.

- Parents can teach children to serve themselves at the table.

- Instruct parents to offer the child a variety of healthy foods and allow the child to choose which ones to eat.

- Instruct parents to modify foods to make them easier and safer for the child to eat.

- Encourage parents to be patient and understanding if the child makes a mess while he learns to feed himself.

- Tell parents that they can encourage the child to eat new foods by offering small portions—perhaps 1 or 2 tablespoons.[6]

- Encourage parents to be positive role models when they offer new foods to the child by eating these foods themselves.

- Caution parents not to pressure the child to eat certain foods or to eat more than she wants.

- Tell parents not to use foods to reward, bribe, or punish the child or to calm, comfort, or entertain him.

- Emphasize that children benefit when parents praise them for their accomplishments and are patient and understanding.

■ Encourage parents to offer dessert as part of the meal. Some desserts (e.g., custard, pudding, fruit, yogurt) make a healthy contribution to the meal.

Food Safety

■ Inform parents that children are at high risk for many foodborne illnesses because their immune and gastrointestinal systems are not fully developed. To reduce the risk of foodborne illness, parents need to follow food safety practices. (See Appendix H: Tips for Promoting Food Safety.)

■ Tell parents to use a highchair or an infant seat when feeding the child.

■ Parents may need instruction about special techniques for positioning, special equipment, or modified utensils for feeding children with special health care needs.

■ Instruct parents to take the following precautions to prevent their children from choking:

Stay with children while they are eating.

Have children sit while eating. Eating while walking or running may cause choking.

Keep things calm at meal and snack times. Overexcitement while eating may cause choking in children.

For children under age 2, foods that may cause choking should be avoided (e.g., hard candy, mini-marshmallows, popcorn, pretzels, chips, spoonfuls of peanut butter, nuts, seeds, large chunks of meat, hot dogs, raw carrots, raisins and other dried fruits, whole grapes).[7]

Children between 2 and 5 may eat these foods if they are modified to make them safer (e.g., cutting hot dogs in quarters lengthwise and then into small pieces, cutting whole grapes in half lengthwise, chopping nuts finely, chopping raw carrots finely or into thin strips, spreading peanut butter thinly on crackers or bread).[7]

■ Caution parents not to let the child eat in the car. If the parent is driving, helping a choking child will be difficult.

Teaching Children About Food

■ Encourage parents to offer a wide variety of healthy foods to the child.

■ Parents can help the child learn about foods from other cultures by offering these foods.

■ Encourage parents to teach the child where foods come from and how foods are grown (e.g., by planting a vegetable garden).

■ Encourage parents to involve the child in food shopping and preparation.

Physical Activity

■ Parents' involvement and enthusiasm have a positive impact on their children's play experiences. Encourage parents to be good role models by playing with their children and participating in physical activity themselves.

■ Suggest that parents plan activities each week to encourage all family members to participate in physical activity.

■ Encourage parents to let the child decide which physical activities the family will do together (e.g., washing the car, raking leaves, walking the dog, hiking, skating, swimming, playing tag).

- Community projects provide opportunities for the entire family to be physically active together (e.g., neighborhood cleanup days, community gardens, food drives).

Oral Health

- Explain to parents that community water fluoridation is a safe and effective way to significantly reduce the risk of early childhood caries. It is best for families to drink fluoridated water; for families that prefer bottled water, a brand in which fluoride is added at a concentration of approximately 0.8 to 1.0 mg/L (ppm) is recommended.[8]

- Inform parents that children require fluoride supplementation if the water is severely deficient in fluoride (i.e., less than 0.3 ppm for children 6 months to 3 years; less than 0.6 ppm for children 3 to 6 years).[8]

- Instruct parents to clean the child's teeth twice a day using a small, soft toothbrush and water. Children can start using fluoridated toothpaste at 2 years of age, but only a pea-size amount. Brushing should be supervised because children ages 2 to 6 are at increased risk for enamel damage if they swallow too much fluoridated toothpaste.

- Explain to parents that limiting the child's consumption of candy, dried fruit, and other foods that stick to the teeth can help prevent early childhood caries.

- Tell parents that to prevent injuries to the child's mouth, teeth, oral tissue, and jaws, they need to use a safety belt when the child is placed in a shopping cart, a child safety seat when the child rides in a car or truck, and baby gates at the top and bottom of stairs.

Nutrition Supervision by Visit

1 YEAR

Health professionals can use the general information in the section Nutrition Supervision Throughout Early Childhood (pp. 63–68), as well as the age-specific information that follows.

Interview Questions

What is Rhonda's feeding routine?

Are you breastfeeding Rhonda? Are you giving her infant formula or milk in a bottle or cup?

What type of infant formula or milk do you feed her?

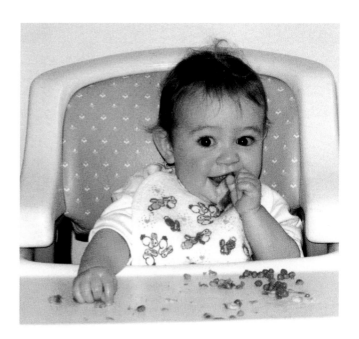

How much fruit juice or how many sweetened drinks (for example, Kool-Aid, fruit punch, or soft drinks) does Rhonda drink? When does she drink them?

Does Rhonda drink from a cup? Does she drink from a bottle now and then? If so, what are your plans for weaning her from the bottle?

What textures of food does Rhonda eat? Does she eat pieces of soft food?

Does she eat meals with the family?

Screening and Assessment

■ Screen the child for iron-deficiency anemia if any of these risk factors are present (see the Iron-Deficiency Anemia chapter):[4]

Was born preterm or with low birthweight

Was fed non–iron-fortified infant formula for more than 2 months

Was fed cow's milk before 12 months of age

Consumes more than 24 oz of cow's milk per day

Is eligible for WIC

Is from a family with low income

Is from a migrant family

Is from a family of recently arrived refugees

Has special health care needs (e.g., takes medications that interfere with iron absorption; has chronic infection, inflammatory disorders, a restricted diet, or extensive blood loss from a wound, an accident, or surgery)

■ Screen the child for lead exposure. (See Appendix E: Screening for Elevated Blood Lead Levels.)

■ Evaluate the child's progress in developing eating skills. Make sure the child

Can bite off small pieces of food.

Can put food in the mouth.

Has an adequate gag reflex.

Can retain food in the mouth (i.e., doesn't immediately swallow).

Can chew food in an up-and-down or rotary motion.

Can use a "pincer grasp" to pick up small pieces of food.

Can drink from a cup.

Nutrition Counseling

■ Encourage parents to give their children opportunities to feed themselves at the family table.

■ Encourage parents to give their children opportunities to develop their eating skills (including chewing and swallowing) by offering a variety of foods.

■ Instruct parents to serve the child beverages in a cup. Children may need help drinking from a cup; however, they may be able to use a covered infant cup by themselves.

■ Encourage parents to serve the child a variety of soft foods.

■ Explain that children are unpredictable in the amount and types of foods they eat, from meal to meal and from day to day. Reassure parents that children usually eat enough food to meet their nutrition needs.

- Instruct parents to offer the child food every 2 to 3 hours, because children's capacity to eat at any one time is limited.

- Explain that children will test limits by asking for certain foods and perhaps by throwing tantrums when refused.

- Reassure parents that they can impose limits on the child's unacceptable mealtime behaviors without controlling the amount or types of foods she eats.

- Instruct parents to clean the child's teeth twice a day using a small, soft toothbrush (without toothpaste) and water.

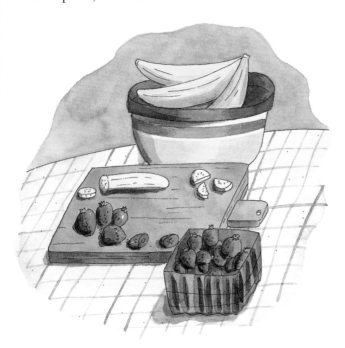

15 MONTHS

Health professionals can use the general information in the section Nutrition Supervision Throughout Early Childhood (pp. 63–68), as well as the age-specific information that follows.

Interview Questions

Are you breastfeeding Christopher? Are you giving him bottles? Milk in a cup? What kind of milk does he drink? How much?

How much fruit juice or how many sweetened drinks (for example, Kool-Aid, fruit punch, or soft drinks) does Christopher drink? When does he drink them?

Which foods does Christopher like to eat? Are there any foods he doesn't like?

Does Christopher eat meals with the family?

Does he ask for food between meals and snacks? If so, how do you handle this?

Does Christopher throw tantrums over food? If so, how do you handle them?

Screening and Assessment

- Screen the child for iron-deficiency anemia if any of these risk factors are present (see the Iron-Deficiency Anemia chapter):[4]

    Was born preterm or with low birthweight

    Was fed non–iron-fortified infant formula for more than 2 months

    Was fed cow's milk before 12 months of age

    Consumes more than 24 oz of cow's milk per day

Is eligible for WIC

Is from a family with low income

Is from a migrant family

Is from a family of recently arrived refugees

Has special health care needs (e.g., takes medications that interfere with iron absorption; has chronic infections, inflammatory disorders, a restricted diet, or extensive blood loss from a wound, accident, or surgery)

Nutrition Counseling

- Instruct parents to offer the child food every 2 to 3 hours, because children's capacity to eat at any one time is limited.

- Emphasize that children benefit from a relaxed atmosphere during meals and snacks. Children should not be rushed, because trying new foods takes time.

- Reassure parents that children will become increasingly skilled at eating a variety of foods.

- Instruct parents to use spoons, cups, and dishes with steep sides (e.g., bowls) to make eating easier for the child.

- Instruct parents to clean the child's teeth twice a day using a small, soft toothbrush (without toothpaste) and water.

18 MONTHS

Health professionals can use the general information in the section Nutrition Supervision Throughout Early Childhood (pp. 63–68), as well as the age-specific information that follows.

Interview Questions

Are you breastfeeding Mia? Are you giving her bottles? Milk in a cup? What kind of milk does she drink? How much?

How much fruit juice or how many sweetened drinks (for example, Kool-Aid, fruit punch, or soft drinks) does Mia drink? When does she drink them?

Which foods does Mia like to eat? Are there any foods she doesn't like?

Does Mia eat meals with the family?

Does she ask for food between meals and snacks? If so, how do you handle this?

Does Mia throw tantrums over food? If so, how do you handle them?

Screening and Assessment

- Use the screening and assessment guidelines in the section Nutrition Supervision Throughout Early Childhood (pp. 63–68).

Nutrition Counseling

- Instruct parents to offer the child food every 2 to 3 hours, because children's capacity to eat at any one time is limited.

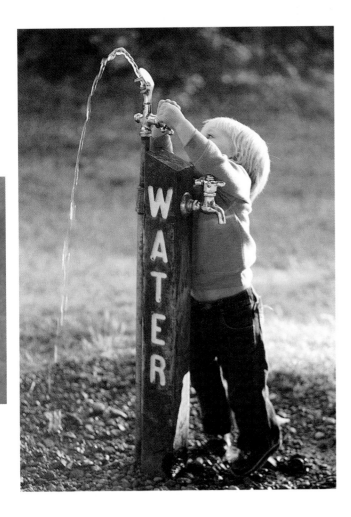

- Encourage parents to give the child opportunities to feed himself at the family table.

- Encourage parents to give the child opportunities to develop her eating skills (including chewing and swallowing) by offering a variety of foods.

- Explain that children need forks and spoons that are designed for them (i.e., those that are smaller and easier to use).

- Instruct parents to clean the child's teeth twice a day using a small, soft toothbrush (without toothpaste) and water.

2 YEARS

Health professionals can use the general information in the section Nutrition Supervision Throughout Early Childhood (pp. 63–68), as well as the age-specific information that follows.

Interview Questions

Has Ricky been weaned from the bottle?

What kind of milk does he drink? How much?

How much fruit juice or how many sweetened drinks (for example, Kool-Aid, fruit punch, or soft drinks) does Ricky drink? When does he drink them?

Which foods does Ricky like to eat? Are there any foods he doesn't like?

Does Ricky eat meals with the family?

Does he eat the same foods as the rest of the family?

What do you do when Ricky does not want to eat or only wants to eat a particular food?

Screening and Assessment

- Screen the child for iron-deficiency anemia if any of these risk factors are present (see the Iron-Deficiency Anemia chapter):[4]

    Consumes a diet low in iron

    Has limited access to food because of poverty or neglect

    Has special health care needs

- Screen the child for lead exposure. (See Appendix E: Screening for Elevated Blood Lead Levels.)

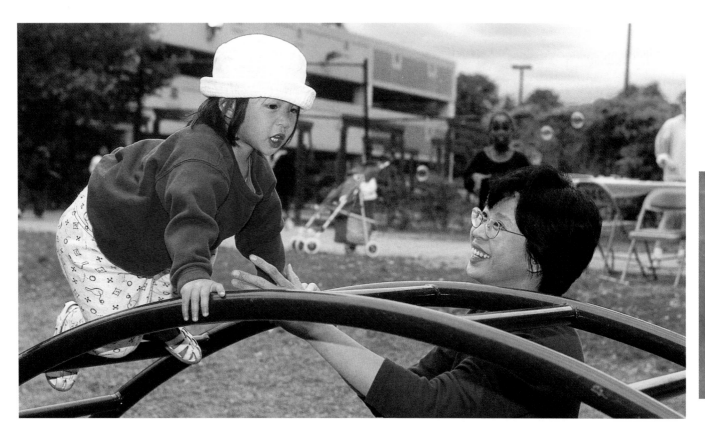

■ Assess the child's risk for familial hyperlipidemia. (See the Hyperlipidemia chapter.)

■ Ask whether the child has regular dental checkups.

Nutrition Counseling

■ Encourage parents to give the child opportunities to develop her eating skills (including chewing and swallowing) by offering a variety of foods.

■ Reassure parents that food jags in children (when children only want to eat a particular food) are common. Smaller servings of the favored food can be offered, along with other foods to ensure that the child eats a variety of healthy foods.

■ Instruct parents to clean the child's teeth twice a day using a small, soft toothbrush and a pea-size amount of fluoridated toothpaste. Brushing should be supervised because children ages 2 to 6 are at increased risk for enamel damage if they swallow too much fluoridated toothpaste.

3 TO 4 YEARS

Health professionals can use the general information in the section Nutrition Supervision Throughout Early Childhood (pp. 63–68), as well as the age-specific information that follows.

Interview Questions

What kind of milk does Felicia drink? How much?

How much fruit juice or how many sweetened drinks (for example, Kool-Aid, fruit punch, or soft drinks) does Felicia drink? When does she drink them?

Which foods does Felicia like to eat? Are there any foods she doesn't like?

Does Felicia eat meals with the family?

How often do you serve snacks? What types of foods do you serve?

Screening and Assessment

■ Screen the child for iron-deficiency anemia if any of these risk factors are present (see the Iron-Deficiency Anemia chapter):[4]

Consumes a diet low in iron

Has limited access to food because of poverty or neglect

Has special health care needs

■ Screen the child for lead exposure. (See Appendix E: Screening for Elevated Blood Lead Levels.)

■ Obtain the child's blood pressure. (See the Hypertension chapter.)

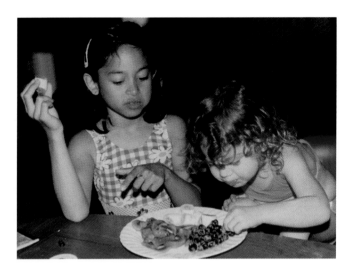

■ Assess the child's risk for familial hyperlipidemia. (See the Hyperlipidemia chapter.)

■ Ask whether the child has regular dental check-ups.

Nutrition Counseling

■ Children become aware of new foods by seeing family and friends enjoying them.

■ Children enjoy learning about new foods by growing, preparing, and talking about them. Sharing stories, drawing pictures, and singing songs related to foods help children become familiar with them.

■ Explain to parents that children 3 years and older need to be taught to brush their teeth twice a day using a small, soft toothbrush and a pea-size amount of fluoridated toothpaste. Brushing should be supervised because children ages 2 to 6 are at increased risk for enamel damage if they swallow too much fluoridated toothpaste.

Table 2. Desired Outcomes for the Child, and the Role of the Family

Child

Educational/Attitudinal	Behavioral	Health
■ Tries new foods ■ Enjoys a variety of healthy foods ■ Enjoys active play	■ Gradually increases variety of foods eaten ■ Eats healthy foods ■ Participates in active play	■ Improves motor skills, coordination, and muscle tone ■ Grows and develops at an appropriate rate ■ Maintains good health

Family

Educational/Attitudinal	Behavioral	Health
■ Understands that each child's growth and development are unique ■ Has a positive attitude toward food ■ Understands the nutrition needs of the growing child and the importance of scheduled healthy meals and snacks ■ Encourages the child to try a variety of healthy foods ■ Understands the importance of modifying foods for the child to make them easier and safer to eat ■ Understands the importance of a healthy lifestyle, including eating healthy foods and participating in regular physical activity	■ Understands that parents are responsible for what, when, and where the child eats, and that the child is responsible for whether to eat and how much ■ Serves developmentally appropriate foods ■ Serves scheduled healthy meals and snacks ■ Offers a variety of foods ■ Eats meals together regularly to ensure optimal nutrition and to facilitate family communication ■ Provides positive role models by eating healthy foods and participating in regular physical activity ■ Uses nutrition programs and food resources if needed ■ Provides safe opportunities for active play	■ Maintains good health

References

1. Birch LL, Fisher JA. 1995. Appetite and eating behavior in children. *Pediatric Clinics of North America* 42(4):931–953.

2. Kleinman RE, ed. 1998. *Pediatric Nutrition Handbook* (4th ed.). Elk Grove Village, IL: American Academy of Pediatrics.

3. Satter EM. 1990. The feeding relationship: Problems and interventions. *Journal of Pediatrics* 117(2, Pt. 2): S181–S189.

4. U.S. Department of Health and Human Services, Centers for Disease Control and Prevention, Epidemiology Program Office. 1998. *Recommendations to Prevent and Control Iron Deficiency in the United States*. Atlanta, GA: U.S. Department of Health and Human Services, Centers for Disease Control and Prevention, Epidemiology Program Office.

5. Satter EM. 1998. *Secrets of Raising a Healthy Eater*. Chelsea, MI: Kelcy Press.

6. U.S. Department of Agriculture, Center for Nutrition Policy and Promotion. 1999. *Tips for Using the Food Guide Pyramid for Young Children 2 to 6 Years Old*. Washington, DC: U.S. Department of Agriculture, Center for Nutrition Policy and Promotion.

7. Graves DE, Suitor CW, Holt KA, eds. 1997. *Making Food Healthy and Safe for Children: How to Meet the National Health and Safety Performance Standards—Guidelines for Out-of-Home Child Care Programs*. Arlington, VA: National Center for Education in Maternal and Child Health.

8. American Dental Association. 1998. *ADA Guide to Dental Therapeutics*. Chicago, IL: ADA Publishing Co.

Suggested Reading

Green M, Palfrey JS, eds. 2000. *Bright Futures: Guidelines for Health Supervision of Infants, Children, and Adolescents* (2nd ed.). Arlington, VA: National Center for Education in Maternal and Child Health.

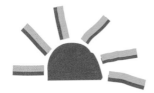

Reducing Distractions During Mealtime

Tyler Mikkelsen, a 22-month-old, is in a home child care facility 5 days a week while his parents work. Like other children his age, Tyler is apprehensive about trying new foods. However, he seems to have a good appetite and his parents have been successful in getting him to try one or two bites of a new food by modeling their own willingness to eat that food.

Tyler's parents are thus surprised when Tyler's child care provider, Fran Eisenberg, asks to speak with them about Tyler's eating. Ms. Eisenberg says that Tyler will not sit down at the table long enough to eat his meal and that Tyler refuses to try new foods and sometimes refuses to eat anything at all. Tyler's parents have not noticed any changes in his eating behaviors at home. They call Sandy Hill, a dietitian, for guidance.

Ms. Hill suggests that Tyler's parents visit Ms. Eisenberg's home when she feeds the children. She says that the mealtime environment at child care may be very different from the environment at home, which may be affecting Tyler's appetite and interest in eating. During their visit, Tyler's parents find that Ms. Eisenberg does not sit down to eat meals with the children. Ms. Eisenberg turns on the television in the kitchen so the children can watch cartoons while they eat. Tyler's parents notice that Tyler is too busy watching the cartoons to pay attention to his food.

Tyler's parents meet with Ms. Eisenberg to discuss the mealtime environment. They tell her that they always eat at the table with Tyler to help him eat and to encourage him to try each food on his plate. They do not turn on the television during mealtimes because it distracts Tyler. Tyler's parents suggest that Ms. Eisenberg join the children at mealtime to provide a familylike atmosphere. They also suggest that the television be turned off.

Ms. Eisenberg agrees to try the changes to see whether Tyler's eating behaviors improve. Two weeks later, she tells Tyler's parents that as a result of the changes, Tyler and the other children in her care are eating better and enjoying mealtimes together.

FREQUENTLY ASKED QUESTIONS
ABOUT NUTRITION IN EARLY CHILDHOOD

■ How can I teach my child healthy eating behaviors?

Be a positive role model—practice healthy eating behaviors yourself.

Eat meals together as a family.

Understand that your child will like or dislike certain foods.

Let your child decide whether to eat and how much.

Offer a variety of healthy foods, and encourage your child to try different ones.

Let your child participate in food shopping and preparation.

Teach your child where foods come from and how foods are grown (for example, plant a garden or visit a farm, orchard, or farmer's market).

Do not use food to reward, bribe, or punish your child.

■ How can I make mealtimes enjoyable?

Serve meals and snacks on a predictable but flexible schedule.

Let your child decide whether to eat and how much.

Be patient and understanding if your child makes a mess while she learns to feed herself.

Use your child's favorite plate, bowl, cup, and eating utensils.

Give your child the opportunity to share the events of the day.

Praise your child for trying new foods and for practicing appropriate behavior at the table.

Create a relaxed setting for meals. Put stresses of the day aside.

Do not insist that your child eat all the foods on her plate before dessert. Consider serving dessert with the meal.

Let your child leave the table when she has finished eating.

■ My 2-year-old's appetite has changed. Should I be worried?

Children grow more slowly from ages 1 to 5. Young children's appetites are usually smaller than those of babies.

Children's appetites change a lot from day to day, even from meal to meal. If your child is energetic and growing, he is probably eating enough.

■ How much should I feed my child?

Children usually eat small portions. Offer small portions, and let your child ask for more if she is still hungry.

Children 2 to 3 need the same number of servings as children 4 to 6, but they may need smaller portions—about $2/3$ of a serving.

By the time your child is 4, she can eat serving sizes similar to those eaten by older family members: $1/2$ cup of fruits or vegetables; $3/4$ cup of juice; 1 slice of bread; 2 to 3 oz of cooked lean meat, poultry, or fish.

Children 2 to 6 need two servings of milk, yogurt, or cheese per day.

■ **My child sometimes dawdles during meals. What can I do?**

It is normal for children to lose interest in an activity, including eating, after a short time. They are also easily distracted. Try to reduce distractions (for example, television) during meals and snacks.

Routines are important to children. Serve scheduled meals and snacks.

■ **What can I do about my picky eater?**

Look at your child's eating over time rather than at each meal. If your child is energetic and growing, he is probably eating enough.

Offer your child food choices and let him decide.

Continue to serve a new food even if your child has rejected it.

Let your child participate in food shopping and preparation.

Do not use food to reward, bribe, or punish your child.

■ **How should I handle food struggles with my child?**

Your child may struggle with you over food in an attempt to make decisions and become independent.

Do not struggle with your child over food. Struggling over food may make her even more determined.

Let your child decide whether to eat and how much.

■ **My child wants to eat only peanut butter sandwiches. What should I do?**

Food jags in children (when children want to eat only a particular food) are common.

Offer smaller servings of the favored food, along with other foods to ensure that your child eats a variety of foods.

Jags rarely last long enough to be harmful. If your child is energetic and growing, he is probably eating enough.

■ **How can I get my child to try new foods?**

Offer small portions of new foods—perhaps 1 or 2 tablespoons—and let your child ask for more.

Encourage your child to try a new food, but don't force her to eat it. She probably won't try new foods if she is tired, irritable, or sick.

Continue to serve a new food even if your child has rejected it. It may take several times before she accepts the food.

Serve your child's favorite foods along with new foods. She may be more willing to try new foods if her favorites are on her plate.

Be a positive role model—eat new foods yourself.

Introduce a new food in a neutral manner. Talk about the food's color, shape, size, aroma, and texture, but don't talk about whether it tastes good.

Make trying new foods appealing by involving your child in shopping and preparing the food.

Be creative. For example, cut foods into various shapes using cookie cutters and create fun names for foods (for example, "little trees" for broccoli).

■ What should I give my child to drink?

Your child may not indicate when he is thirsty. Make sure he drinks water often, especially between meals and snacks.

Your child should consume about 2 cups (16 oz total) of milk per day. Drinking more than this may reduce your child's appetite for other healthy foods.

Children younger then 2 should drink whole milk. Older children can drink 2 percent, low-fat, or skim milk.

Offer juice in small amounts (4 to 8 oz per day). Drinking more than this can reduce your child's appetite for other healthy foods.

Serve your child juice in a cup, not a bottle. Juice served in a bottle can cover your child's teeth with sugar for long periods of time and contribute to early childhood caries (baby bottle tooth decay).

■ How can I help my child, who does not drink milk, get enough calcium?

Serve flavored milk (for example, chocolate or strawberry).

Use dairy foods in recipes (for example, in puddings, milkshakes, soups, casseroles, and cooked cereals).

Serve dairy foods for snacks (for example, cheese, yogurt, and frozen yogurt).

Serve other calcium-rich foods (for example, tofu [if processed with calcium sulfate], broccoli, and turnip greens).

If your child is lactose intolerant, try serving small portions of milk and other dairy foods frequently; milk with a meal or snack; yogurt or lactose-reduced milk; aged hard cheeses (for example, Cheddar, Colby, Swiss, and Parmesan) that are low in lactose; or lactase tablets or drops in the milk.

Serve calcium-fortified foods (for example, orange juice or cereal).

If these strategies don't work, talk to a health professional about giving your child a calcium supplement.

■ Should I give my child a vitamin and mineral supplement?

If your child is growing and eats a variety of healthy foods, she does not need a vitamin and mineral supplement.

If your child does take a vitamin and mineral supplement, keep the bottle out of her reach. The supplement may look like candy, and consuming too many at once can be harmful.

Talk to a health professional if you are considering giving your child a vitamin and mineral supplement.

■ What should I do if my child seems overweight?

If your child is growing, eats healthy foods, and is physically active, you do not need to worry about whether he is overweight.

Let your child know that people come in unique sizes and shapes and that he is loved just as he is. Never criticize your child's size or shape.

If others comment about the size or shape of your child, redirect their comments to your child's other attributes.

Be a role model—practice healthy eating behaviors and participate in regular physical activity.

Focus on gradually changing the entire family's eating behaviors and physical activity practices instead of singling out the overweight child.

Plan family activities that everyone enjoys (for example, hiking, biking, or swimming).

Limit to 1 to 2 hours per day the amount of time your child spends watching television and videotapes and playing computer games.

Serve scheduled meals and snacks.

Do not forbid sweets and desserts. Serve them in moderation.

Never place your child on a diet to lose weight, unless a health professional recommends one for medical reasons and supervises it.

■ How can I help my child like her body?

Be a positive role model—don't criticize your own size or shape or that of others.

Focus on traits other than appearance when talking to your child.

■ Should my child eat low-fat foods?

Skim and low-fat milk are not recommended during the first 2 years, because babies and young children need fat for growth and development.

After 2 years of age, children should gradually eat more low-fat foods. As they begin to consume fewer calories from fat, children need more breads and cereals, fruits and vegetables, low-fat milk, lean meats, and other high-protein foods.

It is important for children to consume enough calories to grow well. When children are very active or having a growth spurt, their energy needs may be higher.

■ How can I prevent my child from choking?

Stay with your child while he is eating.

Have your child sit while eating. Eating while walking or running may cause him to choke on his food.

Keep things calm at meal and snack times. If your child becomes overexcited, he may choke on his food.

Choking can also result when children try to put too much food in their mouths at once.

For children younger than 2, avoid foods that may cause choking (for example, hard candy, mini-marshmallows, popcorn, pretzels, chips, spoonfuls of peanut butter, nuts, seeds, large chunks of meat, hot dogs, raw carrots, raisins and other dried fruits, and whole grapes).

Children ages 2 to 5 may eat these foods if they are modified to make them safer (for example, cutting hot dogs in quarters lengthwise and then into small pieces, cutting whole grapes in half lengthwise, chopping nuts finely, chopping raw carrots finely or into thin strips, and spreading peanut butter thinly on crackers or bread).

Avoid letting your child eat in the car. If he is choking, you won't be able to help him if you are driving.

■ What can I do to make grocery shopping with my child pleasant?

Go shopping when neither you nor your child is hungry.

Make a list in advance to save time at the store.

Use a safety belt when your child rides in a shopping cart.

Bring toys to keep your child busy.

Set up clear rules of behavior (for example, no climbing out of the cart and no asking for candy), and praise your child for following the rules.

Ask your child to help you look for food items.

Talk to your child about what you are buying.

If possible, do not rush your child. Children love to look around and discuss what they see.

■ How can I encourage my child to be more physically active?

Encourage active, spur-of-the-moment play.

Limit to 1 to 2 hours per day the time your child spends watching television and videotapes and playing computer games.

For every hour your child reads, watches television and videotapes, or plays computer games, encourage her to take a 10-minute physical activity break.

Involve your child in family chores (for example, raking leaves or walking the dog).

Plan at least one special physical activity (for example, a hike or bike ride) each week.

Be a positive role model—participate in physical activity yourself.

Play together (for example, play ball, chase, tag, or hopscotch).

Enroll your child in planned physical activities (for example, swimming or dancing lessons or gymnastics).

Work with community leaders to ensure that your child has safe places for participating in physical activity (for example, walking and biking paths, playgrounds, parks, and community centers).

■ What can I expect my child to do as he grows?

1 to 1¹/2 Years

Your child will grasp and release foods with his fingers.

He will be able to hold a spoon but won't be able to use it very well.

He will be able to turn a spoon in his mouth.

He will be able to use a cup but will have difficulty letting go of it.

He will want food that others are eating.

1¹/2 to 2 Years

Your child will eat less.

She will like to eat with her hands.

She will like trying foods of various textures.

She will like routine.

She will have favorite foods.

She will get distracted easily.

2 to 3 Years

Your child will be able to hold a glass.

He will be able to place a spoon straight into his mouth.

He will spill a lot.

He will be able to chew more foods.

He will have definite likes and dislikes.

He will insist on doing things himself.

He will like routine.

He will dawdle during meals.

He will have food jags (when he wants to eat only a particular food).

He will demand foods in certain shapes.

He will like to help in the kitchen.

3 to 4 Years

Your child will be able to hold a cup by its handle.

She will be able to pour liquids from a small pitcher.

She will be able to use a fork.

She will be able to chew most foods.

She will have increased appetite and interest in foods.

She will request favorite foods.

She will like foods in various shapes and colors.

She will choose which foods to eat.

She will be influenced by television.

She will like to imitate the cook.

4 to 5 Years

Your child will be able to use a knife and fork.

He will be able to use a cup well.

He will have an increased ability to feed himself.

He will be more interested in talking than in eating.

He will continue to have food jags.

He can be motivated to eat (for example, by being told "You'll grow up to be tall like your father").

He will like to help prepare food.

He will be interested in where food comes from.

He will be increasingly influenced by peers.

Resources for Health Professionals and Families

Graves DE, Suitor CW, Holt KA, eds. 1997. *Making Food Healthy and Safe for Children: How to Meet the National Health and Safety Performance Standards—Guidelines for Out-of-Home Child Care Programs.* Arlington, VA: National Center for Education in Maternal and Child Health.

Kleinman RE, ed. 1998. *Pediatric Nutrition Handbook* (4th ed.). Elk Grove Village, IL: American Academy of Pediatrics.

Network of the Federal/Provincial/Territorial Group on Nutrition, and National Institute of Nutrition. 1989. *Promoting Nutritional Health During the Preschool Years: Canadian Guidelines.* Ottawa, Ontario, Canada: Network of the Federal/Provincial/Territorial Group on Nutrition, and National Institute of Nutrition.

Satter EM. 1987. *The Popular Young Child: How to Get Your Kid to Eat . . . But Not Too Much.* Palo Alto, CA: Bull Publishing.

U.S. Department of Agriculture, Center for Nutrition Policy and Promotion. 1999. *Tips for Using the Food Guide Pyramid for Young Children 2 to 6 Years Old.* Washington, DC: U.S. Department of Agriculture, Center for Nutrition Policy and Promotion.

U.S. Department of Agriculture, Food and Consumer Service. 1997. *Fun Tips: Using the Dietary Guidelines at Home.* Alexandria, VA: U.S. Department of Agriculture, Food and Consumer Service. Available from http://151.121.3.25/teanut/Resources/funtips.html.

U.S. Department of Agriculture, Food and Nutrition Service. 1999. *Families Who Eat Together . . . Grow Together.* Parent Workshop TEAM Nutrition. Washington, DC: U.S. Department of Agriculture, Food and Nutrition Service.

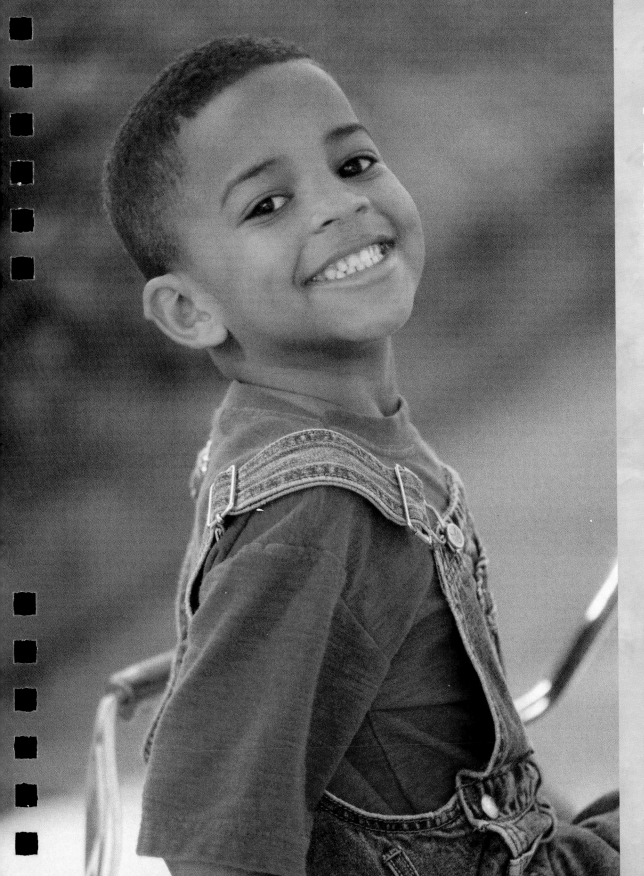

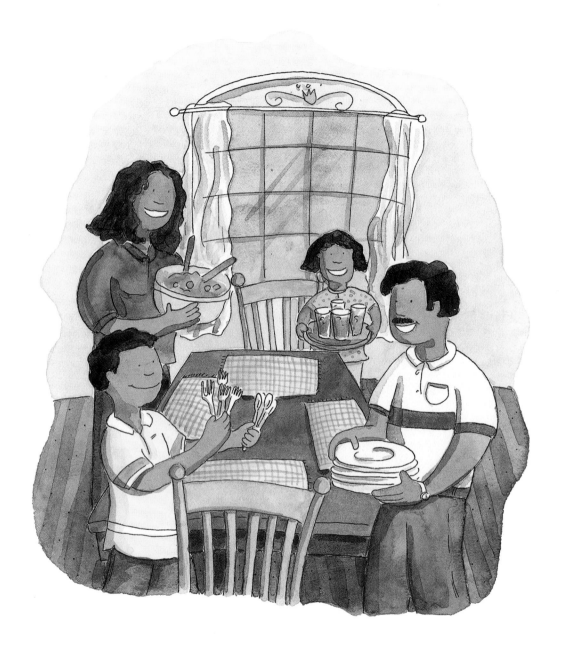

MIDDLE CHILDHOOD

Middle childhood, ages 5 to 10, is characterized by a slow, steady rate of physical growth. However, cognitive, emotional, and social development occur at a tremendous rate.

To achieve optimal growth and development, children need a variety of healthy foods that provide sufficient energy, protein, carbohydrates, fat, vitamins, and minerals. They need three meals per day, plus snacks.

Children benefit greatly from practicing healthy eating behaviors. These behaviors are essential for

- Promoting optimal growth, development, and health.

- Preventing immediate health problems (e.g., iron-deficiency anemia, undernutrition, obesity, eating disorders, dental caries).

- Laying the foundation for lifelong health and reducing the risk of chronic diseases (e.g., cardiovascular disease, type 2 diabetes mellitus, hypertension, some forms of cancer, osteoporosis).

Children also benefit from participating in regular physical activity, which helps reduce the risk of coronary heart disease, hypertension, and colon cancer and helps improve mental health. As children grow and develop, their motor skills increase, giving them more opportunities for participating in physical activity.

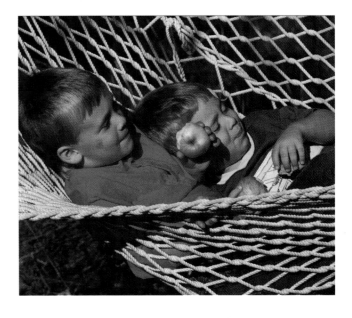

Growth and Physical Development

Middle childhood's slow, steady growth occurs until the onset of puberty, which occurs late in middle childhood or early adolescence. Children gain an average of 7 pounds in weight, an average of 2.5 inches in height, and an average of 2 to 3 cm in head circumference per year. They have growth spurts, which are usually accompanied by an increase in appetite and food intake. Conversely, a child's appetite and food intake decrease during periods of slower growth.

Body composition and body shape remain relatively constant during middle childhood. During preadolescence and early adolescence (9 to 11 years in girls and 10 to 12 years in boys), the percentage of body fat increases in preparation for the growth spurt that occurs during adolescence. This body fat increase occurs earlier in girls than in boys, and the amount of increase is greater in girls. Preadolescents, especially girls, may appear to be "chunky," but this is part of normal growth and development. During middle childhood, boys have more lean body mass per centimeter of height than girls. These differences in body composition become more significant during adolescence.

During middle childhood, children may become overly concerned about their physical appearance. Girls especially may become concerned that they are overweight and may begin to eat less. Parents should be aware of this possibility so that they can reassure their daughters that an increase in body fat during middle childhood is part of normal growth and development and is probably not permanent. Boys may become concerned about their stature and muscle size and strength. Parents should be aware that muscle-building activities (e.g., weightlifting) during this period can be harmful and, in fact, will not build muscle because boys are unable to increase their muscle mass until middle adolescence (although with appropriate physical activity, muscle strength can be improved).

During middle childhood, children's muscle strength, motor skills, and stamina increase. Children acquire the motor skills necessary to perform complex movements, allowing them to participate in a variety of physical activities.

Children begin to lose their primary teeth during middle childhood, and permanent teeth begin to erupt. When children are missing several teeth or are undergoing orthodontic treatment, it may be difficult for them to chew certain foods (e.g., meat). Offering foods that are easier to eat (e.g., crumbled hamburger, chopped meat) can alleviate this problem.

Social and Emotional Development

From ages 5 to 7, children are in the "preoperations" period of development. They describe foods by color, shape, and quantity and classify foods as ones they like and don't like. These children can identify foods that are healthy, but may not know why they are healthy. From ages 7 to 12, children move to the "concrete operations" period of development. These children realize that healthy food has a positive effect on growth and health.

Children in middle childhood begin to develop a sense of self and learn their roles in the family, at school, and in the community. Their ability to feed themselves improves, they can help with meal planning and food preparation, and they can perform tasks related to mealtime (e.g., setting the table). Performing these tasks enables children to contribute to the family, thereby boosting their self-esteem.

During middle childhood, mealtimes take on more social significance and children become more influenced by outside sources (e.g., their peers, the media) regarding eating behaviors and attitudes toward food. In addition, they eat more meals away from home (e.g., at child care facilities, school, and homes of friends and relatives). Their eagerness to eat certain foods and to participate in nutrition programs (e.g., the National School Breakfast and National School Lunch programs) may be based on what their friends are doing. The same principle applies to participation in physical activity. Children may be more interested in activities in which their friends are participating. Participating in physical activity programs and organized sports helps children learn to cooperate with others.

Parents and other family members continue to have the most influence on children's eating behaviors and attitudes toward food. Parents need to make sure that healthy foods are available and decide when to serve them; however, children should decide how much to eat. It is also important for families to eat together in a pleasant environment, allowing time for social interaction.

Healthy Lifestyles

Many children in middle childhood prepare their own breakfasts and snacks. In addition, children may walk to neighborhood stores and fast-food restaurants and purchase foods with their own money. Snacks and fast foods can be high in fat and calories, and their consumption should be limited. Parents can be positive role models by practicing healthy eating behaviors themselves. In addition, parents need to provide guidance to help children make healthy food choices away from home.

Parents are a major influence on a child's level of physical activity. By participating in physical activity (e.g., biking, hiking, playing basketball or baseball) with their children, parents emphasize the importance of regular physical activity—and show their children that physical activity can be fun. Parents' encouragement to be physically active significantly increases a child's activity level.[1]

Teachers also influence a child's level of physical activity. Physical education at school should be provided every day, and enjoyable activities should be offered.

Partnerships with the Community

Middle childhood provides an opportunity for health professionals, families, and communities to teach children about healthy eating behaviors, encourage positive attitudes toward food, and promote regular physical activity. However, there are many barriers. Foods that are high in fat and sugar are readily available, and media messages encourage children to eat them. Children may not have access to the foods they need to stay healthy, as a result of poverty or neglect. Some children do not have opportunities for participating in physical activity, and some live in unsafe neighborhoods.

Children need a variety of foods served in a pleasant environment. Nutrition should be part of the curriculum at school, and child care facilities and school cafeterias should serve a variety of healthy foods that children learn about in the classroom. Federally funded food assistance and nutrition programs can help schools provide children with a substantial part of their daily nutrient requirements. (See Appendix K: Federal Food Assistance and Nutrition Programs.) In addition, community groups, churches and other places of worship, businesses, and others provide food and food vouchers to help hungry or homeless children and families.

Communities need to provide physical activity programs (e.g., at child care facilities, schools, churches and other places of worship, and recreation centers) and safe places for children to play.

Common Nutrition Concerns

During middle childhood, calcium, zinc, and iron are extremely important. Calcium intake by children during this period is declining because milk consumption is decreasing. In addition, fruit and vegetable intake is decreasing. In fact, the intake of fat, saturated fat, and sodium among all children exceeds recommended amounts.[2,3] Consequently, the prevalence of childhood obesity is increasing. In contrast, some children may begin to be overly concerned about their body image during middle childhood, which can lead to eating disorders.[4]

Appendix D: Key Indicators of Nutrition Risk for Children and Adolescents lists the risk factors that can lead to poor nutrition status. If there is evidence that a child is at risk for poor nutrition, further assessment is needed, including a nutritional assessment and/or laboratory tests.

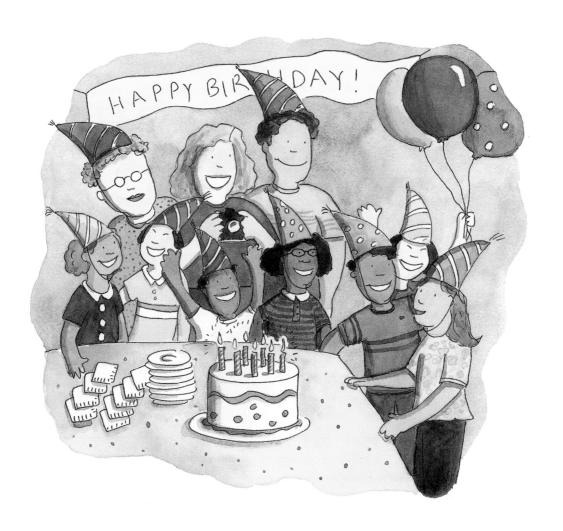

MIDDLE CHILDHOOD NUTRITION SUPERVISION

A child's nutrition status should be evaluated during comprehensive nutrition supervision visits or as part of general health supervision visits. (For more information on health supervision, see *Bright Futures: Guidelines for Health Supervision of Infants, Children, and Adolescents,* listed under Suggested Reading in this chapter.)

Health professionals begin nutrition supervision by gathering information about the child's nutrition status. This can be accomplished by selectively asking key interview questions listed in this chapter or by reviewing a questionnaire filled out by parents before the visit. (See Appendix B: Nutrition Questionnaire for Children.) These methods provide a useful starting point for identifying nutrition concerns.

Health professionals can then use this chapter's screening and assessment guidelines, and nutrition counseling guidelines, to provide families with anticipatory guidance. Interview questions, screening and assessment, and nutrition counseling should be used as appropriate and will vary from visit to visit and from child to child.

To assist health professionals in promoting optimal nutrition that will last a lifetime, desired outcomes for the child and responsibilities for the family are identified in Table 4.

Interview Questions

Eating Behaviors and Food Choices

For the Child

Where did you eat yesterday? At school? At home? At a friend's house?

How often does your family eat meals together?

What do you usually eat and drink in the morning? Around noon? In the afternoon? In the evening? Between meals?

What foods do you eat most often?

What is your favorite food?

Are there special foods you eat during holidays or special occasions?

Are there any foods you won't eat?

Did you drink any milk yesterday? Did you eat other dairy foods (for example, cheese or yogurt)?

Did you eat any fruits yesterday? Vegetables? Did you drink any juice?

For the Parent

Do you think Tran eats healthy foods? Why (or why not)?

What does he usually eat for snacks?

Where does Tran eat snacks? At home? At school? At after-school care? At a friend's house?

Do you have any concerns about his eating behaviors (for example, getting him to drink enough milk)?

Food Resources

For the Child or Parent

Who usually purchases the food for your family? Who prepares it?

Are there times when there is not enough food to eat or not enough money to buy food?

Weight and Body Image

For the Younger Child

How do you feel about the way you look?

Do you feel that you are underweight? Overweight? Just right? Why?

For the Older Child

How much would you like to weigh?

Are you trying to change your weight? If so, why? What are you doing to try to change your weight?

Physical Activity

For the Child

Do you think you are getting enough physical activity? Why (or why not)?

How do you think you can increase your level of physical activity?

How much time do you spend each day watching television and videotapes and playing computer games?

What do you do for fun? Do you ride a bike? Skate? Play basketball or soccer?

Do you take a physical education class at school? If so, what activities do you do in this class?

Do you like physical education? Why (or why not)?

Did you take the President's Council on Physical Fitness and Sports test? If so, how did you do?

Do you participate in sports? If so, which ones?

For the Parent

What type of physical activity does Renae participate in? How often?

Screening and Assessment

■ Measure the child's height and weight, and plot these on a standard growth chart (e.g., the revised Centers for Disease Control and Prevention [CDC]/National Center for Health Statistics [NCHS] growth chart). Deviation from the expected growth pattern (e.g., a major change in growth percentiles on the chart) should be evaluated. This may be normal or may indicate a nutrition problem (e.g., difficulties with eating).

■ Height and weight measurements can be used to indicate nutrition and growth status. Changes in weight reflect a child's short-term nutrient intake and serve as general indicators of nutrition status and overall health. Low height-for-age reflects long-term, cumulative nutrition or health problems.

■ Body mass index (BMI) can be used as a screening tool to determine nutrition status and overall health. Calculate the child's BMI by dividing weight by the square of height (kg/m^2) or by refer-

Table 3. Indicators of Height and Weight Status in Middle Childhood

Indicator	Anthropometric Variable	Cut-Off Values
Stunting (low height-for-age)	Height-for-age	< 3rd percentile
Thinness (low BMI-for-age)	BMI-for-age	< 5th percentile
At risk for overweight	BMI-for-age	≥ 85th percentile, but < 95th percentile
Overweight	BMI-for-age	≥ 95th percentile

Sources: Compiled from World Health Organization[5(p271)] and Himes and Dietz.[6]

ring to a BMI chart. Compare the BMI to the norms listed for the child's sex and age on the chart.

■ Evaluate the appearance of the child's skin, hair, teeth, gums, tongue, and eyes.

■ Obtain the child's blood pressure. (See the Hypertension chapter.)

■ Assess fluoride levels in all sources of water used by the family (including municipal, well, commercially bottled, and home system–processed) to determine the need for fluoride supplementation. If the child is not getting enough fluoride, refer the child to a physician or dentist.

■ Ask whether the child has regular dental checkups.

Stunting

Children whose height-for-age is below the third percentile should be evaluated.[5] Stunting reflects a failure to reach optimum height as a result of poor nutrition or health. Stunting has been reported in children with inadequate food resources, those on highly restricted diets (e.g., diets extremely low in fat), and those with eating disorders or chronic illnesses. The goal is to identify children whose growth is stunted and who may benefit from improved nutrition or treatment of other underlying problems. Most children with low height-for-age are short as a result of genetics, not because their growth is stunted. Children with special health care needs may have low height-for-age because of a genetic disorder, chronic eating problems, altered metabolic rate, malabsorption syndrome, or other conditions. All of these factors should be assessed and interventions implemented to help children reach their potential height.

Thinness

Children with a BMI-for-age below the fifth percentile should be assessed for organic disease and eating disorders. Children may be thin naturally, or they may be thin as a result of a nutritional deficit or chronic disease.

Overweight

Children with a BMI between the 85th and 95th percentiles are at risk for overweight and need further screening. Children with a BMI at or above the 95th percentile for their age and sex are overweight and need an in-depth medical assessment.[3] (See the Obesity chapter.)

Iron-Deficiency Anemia

Children who have a history of iron-deficiency anemia, special health care needs, or low iron intake should be screened for iron-deficiency anemia.[7] (See the Iron-Deficiency Anemia chapter.)

Physical Activity

Assess the child's level of physical fitness by

- Determining how much physical activity the child participates in on a weekly basis.

- Conducting a test (e.g., a modified 3-minute step test) and measuring the child's heart-rate recovery.

- Evaluating how the child's physical fitness compares to national standards (e.g., by reviewing the results of the child's President's Council on Physical Fitness and Sports test).

For physical activity characteristics associated with an increased likelihood of poor nutrition, see Appendix D: Key Indicators of Nutrition Risk for Children and Adolescents. If there is evidence of nutrition risk, further assessment should be done, including a nutrition assessment and/or laboratory tests.

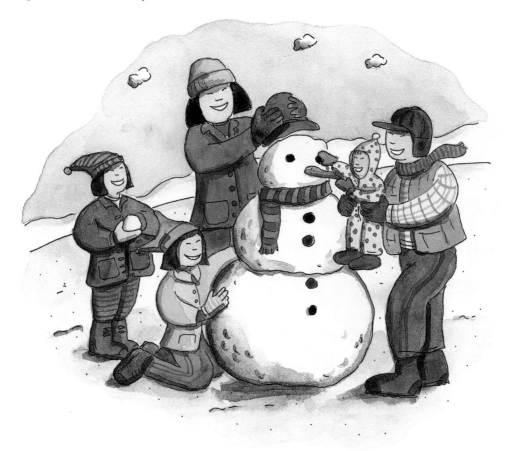

Nutrition Counseling

Health professionals can use the following information to provide anticipatory guidance to parents. Anticipatory guidance provides information on the child's nutrition status and on what to expect as the child enters the next developmental period, and promotes a positive attitude about food and healthy eating behaviors in children. (For additional information on nutrition counseling, see Appendix F: Stages of Change—A Model for Nutrition Counseling, and Appendix G: Strategies for Health Professionals to Promote Healthy Eating Behaviors.)

Physical Development

- Discuss physical development with children and their parents, and the approximate time when they should expect accelerated growth. For girls, this may occur at ages 9 to 11; for boys, this may not occur until about age 12.

- Explain the standard growth chart to children and their parents and how the children compare to others their age. Emphasize that a healthy body weight is based on a genetically determined size and shape rather than on an ideal, socially defined weight. (See Appendix I: Tips for Fostering a Positive Body Image Among Children and Adolescents.)

- Discuss what a healthy weight is. Help children understand that people come in unique sizes and shapes, within a range of healthy body weights. All children need to know they are loved and accepted by their families as they are, regardless of their size and shape.

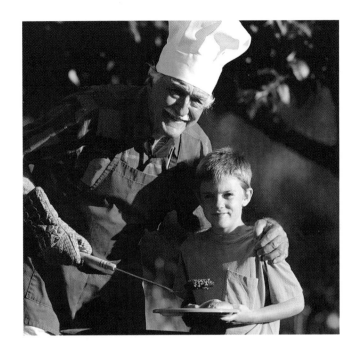

- Explain to older children that some of their peers may start puberty earlier than they do, but that they are still normal.

- Discuss the child's upcoming physical changes and specific concerns.

- Emphasize the importance of eating healthy foods to achieve or maintain a weight appropriate for the child's height and level of physical activity.

- Explain that weight loss should not occur during middle childhood, with the possible exception of the child whose BMI is at or above the 95th percentile.

Eating Behaviors

- Discuss the importance of healthy eating behaviors. Provide guidance to children on increasing the variety of foods they eat and guidance to parents on incorporating new foods into their children's diets.

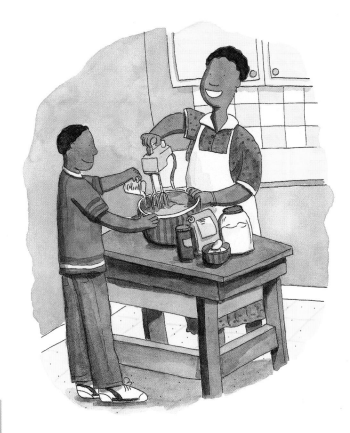

the same amount of kilocalories per day until the beginning of their growth spurts, when calorie needs increase, and 200 to 300 more calories per day may be necessary for very active children.

■ Help children choose healthy snacks rich in complex carbohydrates (e.g., whole grain products, fresh fruits). Encourage families to limit high-fat and high-sugar foods (e.g., chips, candy, soft drinks), as well as foods that increase susceptibility to dental caries. Children in middle childhood cannot consume large amounts of food at one time and therefore need snacks to ensure a healthy diet.

■ Explain to parents that community water fluoridation is a safe and effective way to significantly reduce the risk of dental caries in children. It is best for families to drink fluoridated water; for families that prefer bottled water, a brand in which fluoride is added at a concentration of approximately 0.8 to 1.0 mg/L (ppm) is recommended. Children require fluoride supplementation if their water is severely deficient in fluoride (i.e., less than 0.6 ppm).[8]

Physical Activity

■ Moderate amounts of physical activity are recommended on most, if not all, days of the week. Explain that the child can achieve this level of activity through moderately intense activities (e.g., hiking for 30 minutes) or through shorter, more intense activities (e.g., skating or playing basketball for 15 to 20 minutes).

■ It is critical for children to understand the importance of physical activity. This may encourage them to stay active during adolescence, when physical activity tends to decline.

■ Encourage children to make healthy food choices that are based on the Dietary Guidelines for Americans and the Food Guide Pyramid. (See the Healthy Eating and Physical Activity chapter.)

■ Encourage children to eat healthy meals and snacks. Discuss the importance of eating breakfast, lunch, and dinner. Provide suggestions for packing foods to be eaten away from home, and encourage parents to enroll their children in school breakfast and lunch programs if needed. (See Appendix K: Federal Food Assistance and Nutrition Programs.)

■ Explain that energy requirements remain fairly constant during middle childhood and are influenced by growth, physical activity level, and body composition. Boys and girls need approximately

- Encourage children to find physical activities they enjoy and can incorporate into their daily lives. These activities tend to be continued into adulthood.

- Most elementary schools include physical education in their curricula. Schools that participate in the President's Council on Physical Fitness and Sports program usually conduct testing when children are in middle childhood. Encourage parents to bring the results of their child's fitness testing to discuss positive results as well as suggestions for improvement.

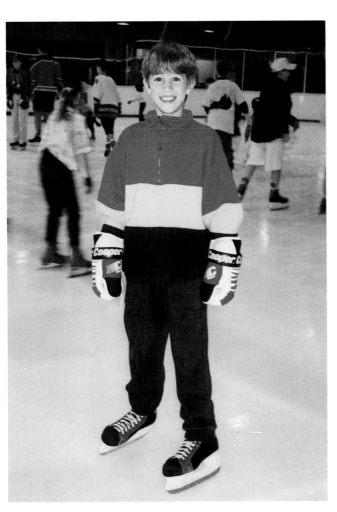

- Encourage parents of children with special health care needs to allow their children to participate in regular physical activity for cardiovascular fitness (within the limits of their medical or physical conditions). Explain that adaptive physical education is often helpful and that a physical therapist can help identify appropriate activities for the child with special health care needs.

- For children who participate in organized sports, adequate fluid intake is very important. Before puberty, children are at increased risk for heat illness because their sweat glands are not fully developed and they cannot cool themselves as well as adolescents can. Encourage parents to make sure that their children drink enough fluids.

- Emphasize the importance of safety equipment (e.g., helmets, pads, mouth guards, goggles) when the child participates in physical activity.

- Encourage children, especially those who are overweight, to reduce sedentary behaviors (e.g., watching television and videotapes, playing computer games).

- If the safety of the environment or neighborhood is a concern, help parents and children find other settings for physical activity.

Substance Use

- Warn parents and children about the dangers of alcohol, tobacco, and other drugs.

- Warn parents and children about the dangers of performance-enhancing products (e.g., protein supplements, anabolic steroids).

Table 4. Desired Outcomes for the Child, and the Role of the Family

Child

Educational/Attitudinal	Behavioral	Health
<ul><li>Understands that healthy eating behaviors and regular physical activity are crucial to growth, development, and health</li><li>Understands the importance of eating a variety of healthy foods and how to increase food variety</li><li>Understands the importance of a healthy diet consisting of 3 meals per day and snacks as needed</li><li>Understands the physical, emotional, and social benefits of regular physical activity and how to increase physical activity level</li><li>Understands that people come in unique body sizes and shapes, within a range of healthy body weights</li></ul>	<ul><li>Consumes a variety of healthy foods</li><li>Makes healthy food choices at and away from home</li><li>Participates in a moderate amount of physical activity on most, if not all, days of the week</li></ul>	<ul><li>Maintains optimal nutrition to promote growth and development</li><li>Achieves nutritional and physical well-being, without signs of iron-deficiency anemia, under-nutrition, obesity, eating disorders, dental caries, or other nutrition-related problems</li><li>Achieves and maintains a healthy body weight and positive body image</li></ul>

(continued)

MIDDLE CHILDHOOD • 5–10 YEARS

Table 4. Desired Outcomes for the Child, and the Role of the Family (continued)

Family

Educational/Attitudinal	Behavioral	Health
■ Understands physical changes that occur with growth and development ■ Understands the relationship between nutrition and short- and long-term health ■ Understands children's eating behaviors and how to increase the variety of foods they eat ■ Understands the importance of a healthy diet consisting of 3 meals per day and snacks as needed ■ Understands that people come in unique body sizes and shapes, within a range of healthy body weights ■ Understands the dangers of unsafe weight-loss methods and knows safe ways to achieve and maintain a healthy weight	■ Provides a positive role model: practices healthy eating behaviors, participates in regular physical activity, and promotes a positive body image ■ Provides a variety of healthy foods at home, limiting the availability of high-fat and high-sugar foods ■ Eats meals together regularly to ensure optimal nutrition and facilitate family communication ■ Provides opportunities for the child to participate in meal planning and food preparation ■ Uses nutrition programs and food resources if needed ■ Participates in regular physical activity with the child	■ Provides developmentally appropriate, healthy foods and modifies them if necessary ■ Helps the child achieve and maintain a healthy weight ■ Provides opportunities and safe places for the child to participate in physical activity

References

1. Epstein LH. 1986. Treatment of childhood obesity. In Brownell KD, Foreyt JP, eds., *Handbook of Eating Disorders*. New York, NY: Basic Books.

2. Johnson RK, Guthrie H, Smiciklas-Wright H, Wang MQ. 1994. Characterizing nutrient intakes of children by sociodemographic factors. *Public Health Reports* 109(3):414–420.

3. Kennedy E, Goldberg J. 1995. What are Americans eating? Implications for public policy. *Nutrition Review* 53(5):111–126.

4. U.S. Department of Health and Human Services, Public Health Service, Office of the Surgeon General. 1988. *Surgeon General's Report on Nutrition and Health*. Washington, DC: U.S. Department of Health and Human Services, Public Health Service, Office of the Surgeon General.

5. World Health Organization. 1995. Physical status: The use and interpretation of anthropometry. Report of a WHO Expert Committee. *World Health Organization Technical Report Series* 854:1–452.

6. Himes JH, Dietz WH. 1994. Guidelines for overweight in adolescent preventive services: Recommendations from an expert committee. *American Journal of Clinical Nutrition* 59(2):307–316.

7. Centers for Disease Control and Prevention, Epidemiology Program Office. 1998. *Recommendations to Prevent and Control Iron Deficiency in the United States*. Atlanta, GA: Centers for Disease Control and Prevention, Epidemiology Program Office.

8. American Dental Association. 1998. *ADA Guide to Dental Therapeutics*. Chicago, IL: ADA Publishing Co.

Suggested Reading

Green M, Palfrey JS, eds. 2000. *Bright Futures: Guidelines for Health Supervision of Infants, Children, and Adolescents* (2nd ed.). Arlington, VA: National Center for Education in Maternal and Child Health.

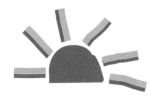

The Importance of Healthy Snacks

By the time Melanie gets home from school around 3:30 p.m., she is very hungry, tired, and cranky.

Melanie Walker is a 6-year-old who has just started first grade. She eats breakfast at home and participates in the school lunch program at her elementary school, where she eats a hot lunch every day at 11:00 a.m. The school does not have a regularly scheduled snack in the afternoon. By the time Melanie gets home from school around 3:30 p.m., she is very hungry, tired, and cranky.

Last year, Melanie attended a morning kindergarten class and spent three afternoons a week at a child care facility. At the time, she was eating breakfast at home, a snack at 9:30 a.m., a hot lunch at 11:30 a.m., and another snack at 3:00 p.m. Melanie didn't seem to be as hungry, tired, or cranky at the end of the afternoon as she is now.

Melanie's parents talk with a nutritionist, Kristin McKee, who suggests that they meet with the teacher and the principal to discuss adding an afternoon snack. Mr. and Mrs. Walker and the parents of other children in Melanie's class share their concerns with the teacher and the principal during an after-school meeting, and the nutritionist shares information on the importance of healthy snacks in children's diets. As a result, the school authorizes a regular afternoon snack for children who eat lunch early.

FREQUENTLY ASKED QUESTIONS ABOUT NUTRITION IN MIDDLE CHILDHOOD

■ **How can our family eat healthy meals together when our schedules are so busy?**

Try eating different meals together (for example, sometimes breakfast and other times lunch or dinner).

Buy healthy ready-to-eat meals from the store or healthy take-out foods from a restaurant.

Have family members share the cooking. Use food preparation and cooking as a family activity.

When your family eats together, use the time to socialize. Avoid distractions. Turn the television off, and don't answer the telephone.

■ **How can I encourage my child to eat breakfast?**

Provide foods that are fast and convenient (for example, bagels, fruit, and yogurt).

Serve foods other than the usual breakfast foods (for example, sandwiches, baked potatoes, and leftovers such as chicken or pasta).

Help your child get organized so that she has time to eat in the morning.

Prepare breakfast the night before.

If your child is in a hurry, suggest that she take some food (for example, fresh fruits or trail mix) to eat on the bus or at school.

If your child is not hungry, offer a breakfast shake (for example, low-fat milk, fruit, and ice mixed in a blender).

■ **How can I get my child to eat more fruits and vegetables?**

Be a positive role model—eat more fruits and vegetables yourself.

Keep a variety of fresh fruits and vegetables in the home.

Keep juice in the refrigerator.

Put a bowl of fruit on the kitchen table or counter.

Eat fruits with meals or for dessert.

Suggest that your child take fruits or vegetables to eat at school.

Wash and cut up fruits and vegetables and keep them in a clear container (so they can be seen easily) in the refrigerator, along with low-fat dip or salsa.

Serve two or more vegetables with dinner (including at least one your child likes). Serve a salad with a choice of dressing.

Use plenty of vegetables in soups, sauces, and casseroles.

Plant a garden.

Offer a variety of fruits and vegetables at meals and snacks, but don't force your child to eat them.

■ **How can I help my child, who does not drink milk, get enough calcium?**

Serve low-fat flavored milk (for example, chocolate or strawberry).

Use low-fat dairy foods in recipes (for example, in puddings, milkshakes, soups, casseroles, and cooked cereals).

Serve low-fat dairy foods for snacks (for example, cheese, yogurt, and frozen yogurt).

Offer unusual dairy foods (for example, yogurt juice drinks and new flavors of low-fat yogurt).

Serve other calcium-rich foods (for example, tofu [if processed with calcium sulfate], broccoli, and turnip greens).

If your child is lactose intolerant, try serving small portions of milk and other dairy foods frequently; milk with a meal or snack; yogurt or lactose-reduced milk; aged hard cheeses (for example, Cheddar, Colby, Swiss, and Parmesan) that are low in lactose; or lactase tablets or drops in the milk.

Serve calcium-fortified foods (for example, orange juice or cereal).

If these strategies don't work, talk to a health professional about giving your child a calcium supplement.

■ How can I teach my child to make healthy food choices away from home?

Encourage your child to make healthy food choices when purchasing food at school, stores, and restaurants, and from vending machines.

Review school and restaurant menus with your child and discuss healthy food choices. Identify on these menus foods that are low in fat and calories.

Encourage your child to eat salads, low-calorie dressings, and broiled or baked meats.

Encourage your child to avoid eating fried foods or to reduce the serving size (for example, by splitting an order of French fries with a friend).

Teach your child to be assertive and to request food modifications (for example, asking the server to "hold the mayonnaise").

■ My child snacks on high-fat and high-sugar foods. What should I do?

Limit the availability of high-fat and high-sugar foods (for example, chips, candy, and soft drinks) at home.

Keep a variety of easy-to-prepare and healthy foods on hand.

Stock up on healthy snack foods (for example, pretzels, baked potato chips, popcorn, juice, fruit, vegetables, low-fat granola bars, and yogurt).

Wash and cut up vegetables and keep them in a clear container (so they can be seen easily) in the refrigerator, along with low-fat dip or salsa.

Put a bowl of fruit on the kitchen table or counter.

Encourage your child to make healthy food choices when purchasing food at school, stores, and restaurants, and from vending machines.

■ My child has become a vegetarian. Should I be concerned?

With careful planning, a vegetarian lifestyle can be healthy and meet the needs of a growing child.

A vegetarian diet that includes dairy foods and eggs usually provides adequate nutrients; however, your child may need to take an iron supplement.

Vegans are strict vegetarians who don't eat any animal products, including dairy foods, eggs, or fish. They may need additional calcium, vitamin B_{12}, and vitamin D, which can be provided by fortified foods and supplements.

Instead of always preparing separate vegetarian meals for your child, occasionally fix vegetarian meals for the whole family.

Ask a dietitian or nutritionist to help you plan healthy meals.

■ What should I do if my child seems overweight?

If your child is growing, eats healthy foods, and is physically active, you do not need to worry about whether he is overweight.

Let your child know that people come in unique sizes and shapes and that he is loved just as he is. Never criticize your child's size or shape.

If others comment about the size or shape of your child, redirect their comments to your child's other attributes.

Be a positive role model—practice healthy eating behaviors and participate in regular physical activity yourself.

Focus on gradually changing the entire family's eating behaviors and physical activity practices instead of singling out the overweight child.

Plan family activities that everyone enjoys (for example, hiking, biking, or swimming).

Limit to 1 to 2 hours per day the amount of time your child watches television and videotapes and plays computer games.

Serve scheduled meals and snacks.

Reduce the amount of high-fat and high-sugar foods in your family's meals and snacks.

Do not forbid sweets and desserts. Serve them in moderation.

Never place your child on a diet to lose weight, unless a health professional recommends one for medical reasons and supervises it.

■ How can I help my child like her body?

Children are very sensitive about comments related to their appearance. Do not criticize your child's size or shape.

Be a positive role model—don't criticize your own size or shape or that of others.

Focus on traits other than appearance when talking to your child.

Discuss how the media affects your child's body image.

■ How can I help my underweight child gain weight?

Limit the quantity of beverages your child drinks between meals if his appetite is being affected.

Serve an after-school snack, and encourage your child to eat a midmorning snack at school, if possible. Limit snacks close to mealtimes if snacking is affecting his appetite.

Involve your child in meal planning and food preparation.

Continue to offer foods even if your child has refused to eat them before. Your child is more likely to accept these foods after they have been offered several times.

■ How can I encourage my child to be more physically active?

Encourage active, spur-of-the-moment physical activity and play.

Limit to 1 to 2 hours per day the time your child spends watching television and videotapes and playing computer games.

For every hour your child reads, watches television and videotapes, or plays computer games, encourage her to take a 10-minute physical activity break.

Involve your child in family chores (for example, raking leaves or walking the dog).

Plan at least one special physical activity (for example, taking a hike or riding a bike) each week.

Incorporate physical activities with your child into your daily life (for example, by using the stairs instead of taking an elevator or escalator, and by walking or riding a bike instead of driving a car).

Be a positive role model—participate in physical activity yourself.

Participate in physical activity together (for example, by playing ball or going biking, dancing, or skating).

Enroll your child in planned physical activities (for example, swimming, martial arts, gymnastics, or dancing).

Work with community leaders to ensure that your child has safe places for participating in physical activity (for example, walking and biking paths, playgrounds, parks, and community centers).

■ What are common symptoms of eating disorders?

Common symptoms of anorexia nervosa are as follows:

Excessive weight loss in a short period of time

Continuation of dieting although thin

Dissatisfaction with appearance; belief that body is fat, even though severely thin

Loss of menstrual period

Unusual interest in certain foods and development of unusual eating rituals

Eating in secret

Obsession with exercise

Depression

Common symptoms of bulimia nervosa are as follows:

Loss of menstrual period

Unusual interest in certain foods and development of unusual eating rituals

Eating in secret

Obsession with exercise

Depression

Binge-eating

Binge-eating with no noticeable weight gain

Vomiting or laxative use

Disappearance into bathroom for long periods of time (e.g., to induce vomiting)

Alcohol or drug abuse

Resources for Health Professionals and Families

Clark N. 1996. *Nancy Clark's Sports Nutrition Guidebook* (2nd ed.). Champaign, IL: Human Kinetics.

Dietz WH, Stern L, eds. 1999. *Guide to Your Child's Nutrition: Making Peace at the Table and Building Healthy Eating Habits for Life.* Elk Grove Village, IL: American Academy of Pediatrics.

National Institutes of Health, National Institute of Diabetes and Digestive and Kidney Diseases. 1997. *Helping Your Overweight Child.* Bethesda, MD: National Institutes of Health, National Institute of Diabetes and Digestive and Kidney Diseases.

National Institutes of Health, National Institute of Mental Health. 1993. *Eating Disorders.* Bethesda, MD: National Institutes of Health, National Institute of Mental Health.

Nissenberg SK, Bogle ML, Wright AC. 1995. *Quick Meals for Healthy Kids and Busy Parents.* Minneapolis, MN: Chronimed Publishing.

Storlie J. 1997. *Snacking Habits for Healthy Living.* Minneapolis, MN: Chronimed Publishing.

Tamborlane WV, Weiswasser JZ, Held NA, Fung T. 1997. *The Yale Guide to Children's Nutrition.* New Haven, CT: Yale University Press.

Trahms CM, Pipes PL. 1997. *Nutrition in Infancy and Childhood* (6th ed.). New York, NY: WCB/McGraw-Hill.

U.S. Department of Agriculture, Food and Consumer Service. 1997. *Fun Tips: Using the Dietary Guidelines at Home.* Alexandria, VA: U.S. Department of Agriculture, Food and Consumer Service. In USDA's Team Nutrition [Web site]. Cited August 13, 1999; available at http://151.121.3.25/teanut/Resources/funtips.html or by written request to USDA's Team Nutrition, 3101 Park Center Drive, Room 1010, Alexandria, VA 22302.

Warner P. 1996. *Healthy Snacks for Kids.* San Leandro, CA: Bristol Publishing Enterprises.

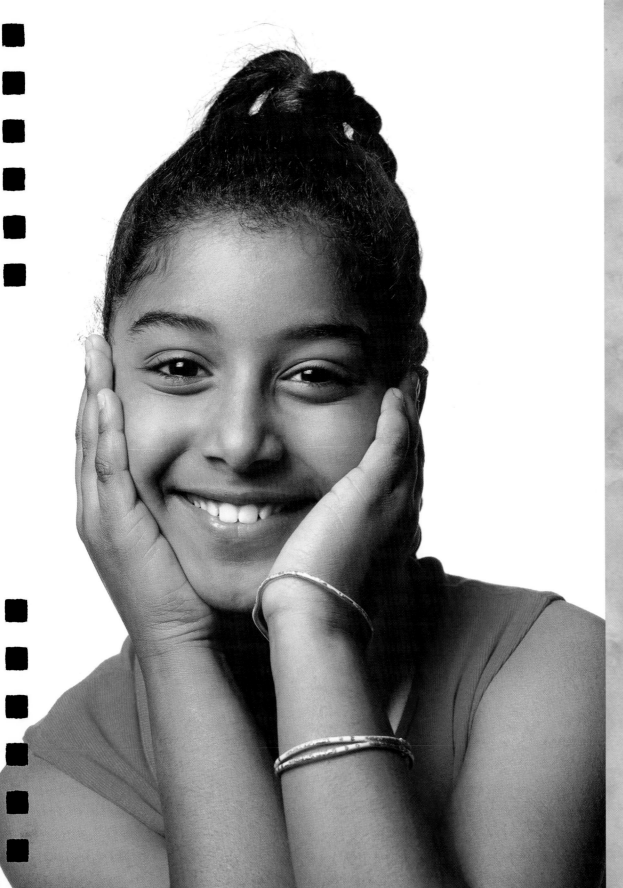

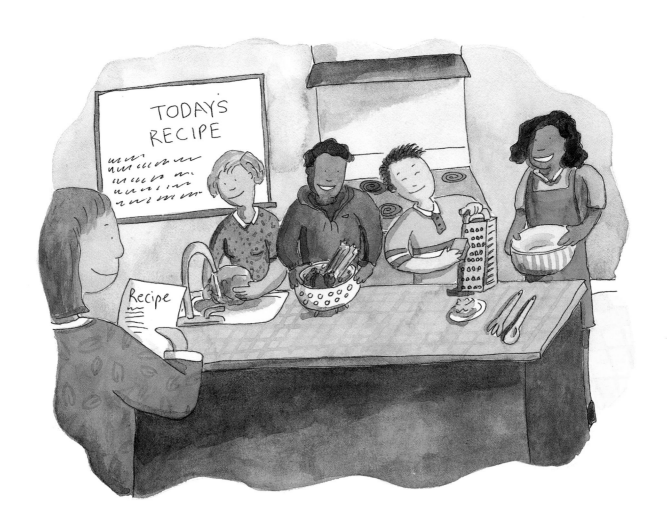

ADOLESCENCE

A dolescence (ages 11 to 21), the transition between childhood and adulthood, is one of the most dynamic periods of human development. Adolescence is characterized by dramatic physical, cognitive, social, and emotional changes. These changes, along with adolescents' growing independence, search for identity, concern with appearance, need for peer acceptance, and active lifestyle, can significantly affect their eating behaviors and nutrition status.

Rapid physical growth creates an increased demand for energy and nutrients. Practicing healthy eating behaviors during adolescence is essential for

- Promoting optimal growth, development, and health.

- Preventing immediate health problems (e.g., iron-deficiency anemia, undernutrition, obesity, eating disorders, dental caries).

- Laying the foundation for lifelong health and reducing the risk of chronic diseases (e.g., cardiovascular disease, type 2 diabetes mellitus, hypertension, some forms of cancer, osteoporosis).

The period of adolescence is divided into three stages. Early adolescence, ages 11 to 14, includes pubertal and cognitive changes. Middle adolescence, ages 15 to 17, is a time of increased independence and experimentation. During late adolescence, ages 18 to 21, adolescents make important personal and vocational decisions. These stages provide a useful context for understanding the eating behaviors and body-image issues of adolescents, as well as a frame-

work for providing adolescents with the information they need to practice healthy eating behaviors and participate in regular physical activity.

Growth and Physical Development

The phenomenal growth that occurs during adolescence is second only to the growth that occurs during the first year of life, and it increases the body's demand for energy and nutrients. Nutrition needs are greater during adolescence than at any other time in the life cycle. During this period, adolescents achieve the final 15 to 20 percent of their adult height, gain 50 percent of their adult body weight, and accumulate up to 40 percent of their adult skeletal mass.[1] Nutrient needs parallel the rate of growth, with the greatest demands occurring during the peak period of growth (sexual maturity rating [SMR] 2 to 3 in females and 3 to 4 in males). For females, most physical growth is completed by about 2 years after menarche. (The mean age of menarche is 12.5 years.) Males begin puberty about 2 years later than females, and they typically experience their major growth spurt and increase in muscle mass during middle adolescence.

Nutrition and physical activity are major determinants of adolescents' energy levels and influence growth and body composition. Inadequate nutrition can delay sexual maturation, slow or stop linear growth, and compromise peak bone mass. Practicing healthy eating behaviors and participating in regular physical activity can help adolescents achieve normal body weight and body composition, thereby reducing their risk of obesity.

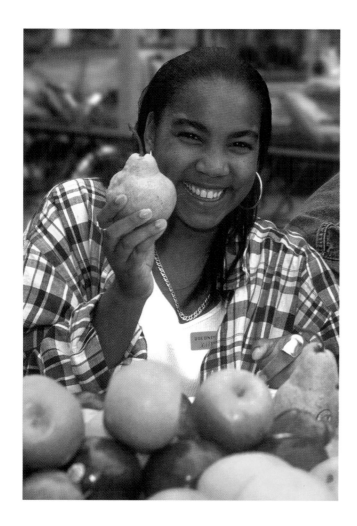

The changes associated with puberty affect adolescents' satisfaction with their appearance. For males, the increased size and muscular development that come with physical maturation usually improve their body image. However, physical maturation among females may lead to dissatisfaction with their bodies, which may result in weight concerns and dieting.

Anticipatory guidance can help prepare adolescents and their parents for changes associated with puberty and help adolescents develop a positive body image. Because adolescents usually are interested in their growth and development, this period is a key opportunity for health professionals to discuss the importance of healthy eating behaviors, regular physical activity, and a positive body image.

Cognitive capacities increase dramatically during adolescence. During early adolescence, adolescents have a growing capacity for abstract thought, but their thinking still tends to be concrete and oriented toward the present. During middle adolescence, they become more capable of problem solving and abstract and future-oriented thinking. During late adolescence, they continue to refine their ability to reason logically and solve problems. The cognitive changes that occur during adolescence should facilitate nutrition supervision, because adolescents are beginning to reflect on their behavior and understand its consequences.

Undernutrition compromises cognitive development, which affects learning, concentration, and school performance. Conversely, eating breakfast improves cognitive performance and learning.[2]

Social and Emotional Development

Developing an identity and becoming an independent young adult are central to adolescence. Because foods can have symbolic meanings, adolescents may use them to establish individuality and express their identity.

Experimentation and idealism are common during middle adolescence. Adolescents may adopt certain eating behaviors (e.g., vegetarianism) to explore various lifestyles or to show concern for the environment. Adolescents are usually interested in new foods, including those from different cultures and ethnic groups.

Adolescents may try fad diets—and underestimate the health risks associated with them. The social pressure to be thin and the stigma of obesity can lead to unhealthy eating behaviors and a poor body image. Health professionals can help adolescents practice healthy eating behaviors, participate in regular physical activity, and develop a positive body image. (See Appendix I: Tips for Fostering a Positive Body Image Among Children and Adolescents.)

Adolescents spend a lot of time with their friends, and peer influence and group conformity are important. They may eat certain foods to demonstrate loyalty to their friends. Because much of their physical activity occurs in group settings, adolescents' participation in physical activity may be influenced by peers.

Healthy Lifestyles

As adolescents strive for independence, they begin to spend more time away from home and thus eat more meals and snacks away from home. Although parents cannot control what their adolescents eat when they are away from home, they can make sure that healthy foods are available at home.

Many adolescents walk or drive to neighborhood stores and fast-food restaurants and purchase foods with their own money. Snacks and fast foods can be high in fat and calories, and their consumption should be limited. Parents can be positive role models by practicing healthy eating behaviors themselves. In addition, parents need to provide guidance to help adolescents make healthy food choices away from home.

Parents are a major influence on an adolescent's level of physical activity. By participating in physical activity (e.g., biking, playing basketball or baseball) with their adolescents, parents emphasize the importance of regular physical activity—and show their adolescents that physical activity can be fun. Parents' encouragement to be physically active significantly increases an adolescent's activity level.

Teachers also influence an adolescent's level of physical activity. Physical education at school should be provided every day, and enjoyable activities should be offered.

Partnerships with the Community

Healthy eating behaviors and regular physical activity promote the nutrition status of adolescents. Partnerships among health professionals, families, and communities are integral to developing nutrition and physical activity programs.

Schools can play a significant role in promoting healthy eating behaviors among adolescents. Nutrition education should be integrated within a comprehensive school health-education program for adolescents.[3,4] School cafeterias can reinforce what is taught in the classroom by providing healthy foods. Other foods sold at school (e.g., in vending machines, at sports events, for fund-raising) should be healthy. Federally funded food assistance and nutrition programs can help schools provide adolescents with a substantial part of their daily nutrition requirements. (See Appendix K: Federal Food Assistance and Nutrition Programs.) In addition, community groups, churches and other places of worship, and businesses can provide food and food vouchers to help hungry or homeless adolescents and families.

Common Nutrition Concerns

As a group, adolescents do not adhere to the Dietary Guidelines for Americans.[5] Intake of certain vitamins (folate, vitamin A, vitamin B_6) and minerals (iron, calcium, zinc) is inadequate, particularly among adolescents from families with low incomes and among adolescent females. Excessive intake of fat, saturated fat, cholesterol, sodium, and sugar are common in adolescents and occur at all income levels, in all racial/ethnic groups, and in both sexes. Over the past decade, obesity has become more prevalent among adolescents of both sexes.[6] Even so, hunger may be of concern among adolescents from families with low incomes.

Other nutrition concerns for adolescents include low intake of fruits, vegetables, and calcium-rich foods; high soft-drink consumption; unsafe weight-loss methods; iron-deficiency anemia (in females); eating disorders; hyperlipidemia; and low levels of physical activity.[3] Nutrition problems may also occur as a result of neglect, abuse, pregnancy, disabilities, chronic health conditions, or substance abuse.

Appendix D: Key Indicators of Nutrition Risk for Children and Adolescents lists the risk factors that can lead to poor nutrition status. If there is evidence that an adolescent is at risk for poor nutrition, further assessment is needed, including a nutritional assessment and/or laboratory tests.

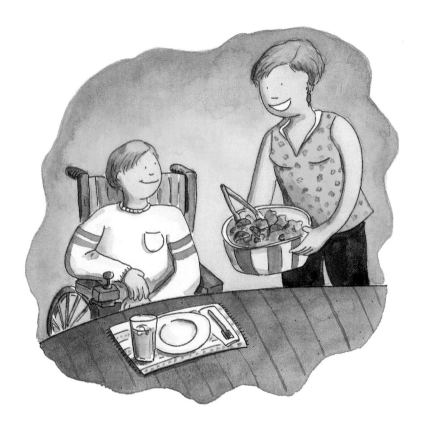

weight before puberty to 20 to 25 percent at the end of puberty).

■ Adolescent males have a mild weight gain before their growth spurt (i.e., increase in height), which occurs at 9 to 13 years of age. In addition, their percentage of body fat decreases during their growth spurt (sexual maturity rating 3 to 4). After puberty, their percentage of body fat increases, and by age 18, it is about 15 to 18 percent of their body weight. Reassure adolescent males and their parents that fat gain is normal and will probably level off during the upcoming growth spurt.

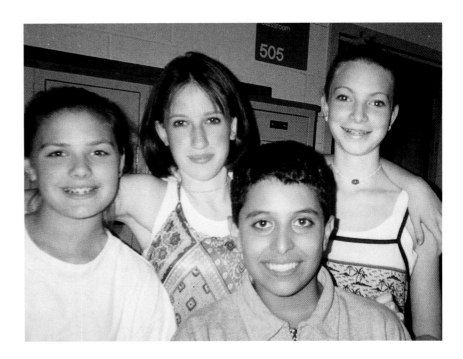

Eating Behaviors

■ Energy requirements increase greatly during adolescence and are influenced by growth status, physical activity level, and body composition. Adolescent males need about 2,500 to 3,000 calories per day, and females need about 2,000 calories per day. An additional 600 to 1,000 calories per day are needed if the adolescent is involved in vigorous physical activity. Reassure adolescents and their parents that it is normal for adolescents to eat more during growth spurts.

■ Discuss healthy eating behaviors, ways to achieve them, and the importance of not skipping meals. Encourage healthy food choices that are based on the Dietary Guidelines for Americans and the Food Guide Pyramid. (See the Healthy Eating and Physical Activity chapter.)

■ The quality of the diet often decreases from childhood through adolescence because adolescents are more independent and make their own food choices. Encourage adolescents to practice healthy eating behaviors. Encourage parents to provide a variety of healthy foods at home and to make family mealtimes a priority.

■ Encourage adolescents to choose healthy foods when eating away from home.

■ Many adolescent females begin to diet after the onset of puberty. Early-maturing females are more likely to diet shortly after puberty than those who mature later. Overweight adolescent females are also more likely to diet and use unhealthy weight-loss practices. Discuss safe and healthy ways to achieve and maintain a healthy body weight. Promote a positive body image and encourage regular physical activity.

■ Explain that community water fluoridation is a safe and effective way to significantly reduce the risk of dental caries in adolescents. It is best for families to drink fluoridated water; for families that prefer bottled water, a brand in which fluoride is added at a concentration of approximately 0.8 to 1.0 mg/L (ppm) is recommended. Adolescents up to 16 years require fluoride supplementation if their water is severely deficient in fluoride (less than 0.6 ppm).[10]

Weight and Body Image

■ Help the adolescent build a positive body image by explaining that people come in unique sizes and shapes, within a range of healthy body weights. Adolescents need to know that they are loved and accepted as they are, regardless of their size and shape. (See Appendix I: Tips for Fostering a Positive Body Image Among Children and Adolescents.)

■ Discuss healthy and safe ways for adolescents to achieve and maintain a healthy weight (e.g., by practicing healthy eating behaviors and participating in regular physical activity). Emphasize that weight reduction through dieting or other means is not advisable for adolescents, who are still growing.

Physical Activity

■ Moderate amounts of physical activity are recommended on most, if not all, days of the week. Explain that the adolescent can achieve this level

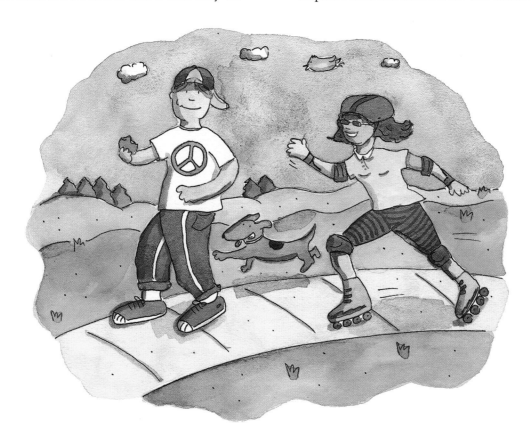

of activity through moderately intense activities (e.g., hiking for 30 minutes) or through shorter, more intense activities (e.g., jogging or playing basketball for 15 to 20 minutes).

- Participation in physical activity declines dramatically during early adolescence, especially in females. Help adolescents incorporate regular physical activity into their daily lives (e.g., through physical education at school and activities with family and friends).

- Encourage adolescents to drink plenty of fluids when they are physically active.

- Emphasize the appropriate use of safety equipment (e.g., helmets, pads, mouth guards, goggles) when the adolescent participates in physical activity.

- Encourage adolescents, especially those who are overweight, to reduce sedentary behaviors (e.g., watching television and videotapes, playing computer games).

- If the safety of the environment or neighborhood is a concern, help adolescents find other settings for physical activity.

Substance Use

- Warn adolescents about the dangers of using alcohol, tobacco, and other drugs.

- Warn adolescents about the dangers of using performance-enhancing products (e.g., protein supplements, anabolic steroids).

Middle Adolescence: 15 to 17 Years

Physical Development

- Explain the standard growth chart to adolescents, and show them how they compare to other adolescents their age. Discuss their upcoming physical changes and specific concerns. Emphasize that a healthy body weight is based on a genetically determined size and shape rather than on an ideal, socially defined weight. (See Appendix I: Tips for Fostering a Positive Body Image Among Children and Adolescents.)

- Help adolescents understand and accept normal physical changes (e.g., weight changes; the widening of females' hips and fat accumulation in their bodies; the large variation in height, weight, and growth rates among adolescents).

- Reassure late-maturing adolescent males that they are normal. Use charts that plot height velocity by age and sexual maturity rating to ease their concerns.

Eating Behaviors

- Energy requirements increase greatly during adolescence and are influenced by growth status, physical activity level, and body composition. Adolescent males need about 2,500 to 3,000 calories per day, and females need about 2,000 calories per day. An additional 600 to 1,000 calories per day are needed if the adolescent is involved in vigorous physical activity. Reassure adolescents and their parents that it is normal for adolescents to eat more during growth spurts.

- Discuss healthy eating behaviors, ways to achieve them, and the importance of not skipping meals. Encourage healthy food choices that are based on

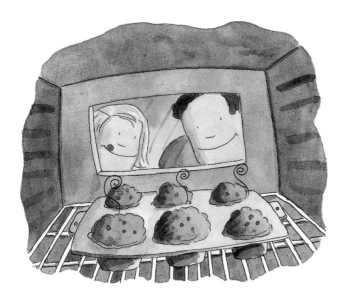

the Dietary Guidelines for Americans and the Food Guide Pyramid. (See the Healthy Eating and Physical Activity chapter.)

■ The quality of the diet often decreases from childhood through adolescence because adolescents are more independent and make their own food choices. Encourage adolescents to practice healthy eating behaviors. Encourage parents to provide a variety of healthy foods at home and to make family mealtimes a priority.

■ Encourage adolescents to choose healthy foods when eating away from home.

■ Explain that community water fluoridation is a safe and effective way to significantly reduce the risk of dental caries in adolescents. It is best for families to drink fluoridated water; for families that prefer bottled water, a brand in which fluoride is added at a concentration of approximately 0.8 to 1.0 mg/L (ppm) is recommended. Adolescents up to 16 years require fluoride supplementation if their water is severely deficient in fluoride (less than 0.6 ppm).[10]

Weight and Body Image

■ Help the adolescent build a positive body image by explaining that people come in unique sizes and shapes, within a range of healthy body weights. Adolescents need to know that they are loved and accepted as they are, regardless of their size and shape. (See Appendix I: Tips for Fostering a Positive Body Image Among Children and Adolescents.)

■ Discuss healthy and safe ways for adolescents to achieve and maintain a healthy weight (e.g., by practicing healthy eating behaviors and participating in regular physical activity). Emphasize that weight reduction through dieting or other means is not advisable for adolescents, who are still growing.

Physical Activity

■ Moderate amounts of physical activity are recommended on most, if not all, days of the week. Explain that the adolescent can achieve this level of activity through moderately intense activities (e.g., hiking for 30 minutes) or through shorter, more intense activities (e.g., jogging or playing basketball for 15 to 20 minutes).

■ Encourage adolescents to drink plenty of fluids when they are physically active.

■ Emphasize the appropriate use of safety equipment (e.g., helmets, pads, mouth guards, goggles) when the adolescent participates in physical activity.

■ Encourage adolescents, especially those who are overweight, to reduce sedentary behaviors (e.g., watching television and videotapes, playing computer games).

- If the safety of the environment or neighborhood is a concern, help adolescents find other settings for physical activity.

Substance Use

- Warn adolescents about the dangers of using alcohol, tobacco, and other drugs.

- Adolescent males, especially those who mature late, may be interested in using protein supplements or anabolic steroids to try to build muscle mass. Discourage the use of these products.

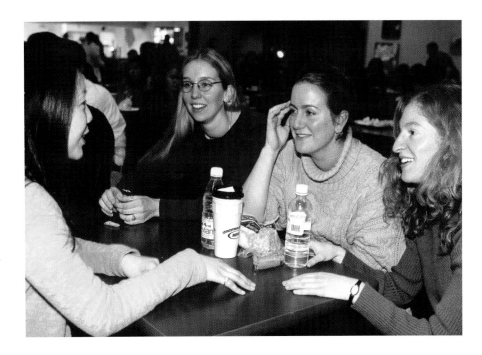

Late Adolescence: 18 to 21 Years

Physical Development

- Explain the standard growth chart to adolescents, and show them how they compare to other adolescents their age. Discuss any specific concerns. Emphasize that a healthy body weight is based on a genetically determined size and shape rather than on an ideal, socially defined weight. (See Appendix I: Tips for Fostering a Positive Body Image Among Children and Adolescents.)

Eating Behaviors

- Energy requirements increase greatly during adolescence and are influenced by growth status, physical activity level, and body composition. Adolescent males need about 2,500 to 3,000 calories per day, and females need about 2,000 calories per day. An additional 600 to 1,000 calories per day are needed if the adolescent is involved in vigorous physical activity.

- Discuss healthy eating behaviors, ways to achieve them, and the importance of not skipping meals. Encourage healthy food choices that are based on the Dietary Guidelines for Americans and the Food Guide Pyramid. (See the Healthy Eating and Physical Activity chapter.)

- Encourage parents to provide a variety of healthy foods at home and to make family mealtimes a priority.

- As older adolescents prepare to leave home for college or to join the workforce or military, they become responsible for making their own food choices. Discuss how the adolescent can make healthy food choices and participate in regular physical activity when living away from home. Parents should be aware of changes in their adolescent's eating behaviors and weight.

- Explain that community water fluoridation is a safe and effective way to significantly reduce the risk of dental caries in adolescents. It is best for families to drink fluoridated water; for families that prefer bottled water, a brand in which fluoride is added at a concentration of approximately 0.8 to 1.0 mg/L (ppm) is recommended.[10]

Weight and Body Image

- Help the adolescent build a positive body image by explaining that people come in unique sizes and shapes, within a range of healthy body weights. Adolescents need to know that they are loved and accepted as they are, regardless of their size and shape. (See Appendix I: Tips for Fostering a Positive Body Image Among Children and Adolescents.)

- Discuss healthy and safe ways for adolescents to achieve and maintain a healthy weight (e.g., by practicing healthy eating behaviors and participating in regular physical activity).

- Because pubertal development is complete at this stage, help adolescents accept their body size and shape. (See Appendix I: Tips for Fostering a Positive Body Image Among Children and Adolescents.)

Physical Activity

- Moderate amounts of physical activity are recommended on most, if not all, days of the week. Explain that the adolescent can achieve this level of activity through moderately intense activities (e.g., hiking for 30 minutes) or through shorter, more intense activities (e.g., jogging or playing basketball for 15 to 20 minutes).

- Many adolescents become less active as they approach adulthood. Discuss how adolescents can incorporate physical activity into their daily lives (e.g., by using the stairs instead of taking the elevator or escalator) and participating in physical activities with friends and family (e.g, walking, running, hiking, biking).

- Encourage adolescents to drink plenty of fluids when they are physically active.

- Emphasize the appropriate use of safety equipment (e.g., helmets, pads, mouth guards, goggles) when the adolescent participates in physical activity.

- Encourage adolescents, especially those who are overweight, to reduce sedentary behaviors (e.g., watching television and videotapes, playing computer games).

- If the safety of the environment or neighborhood is a concern, help adolescents find other settings for physical activity.

Substance Use

- Warn adolescents about the dangers of using alcohol, tobacco, and other drugs.

- Adolescent males may be interested in using protein supplements or anabolic steroids to try to build muscle mass. Discourage the use of these products.

Table 6. Desired Outcomes for the Adolescent, and the Role of the Family

Adolescent

Educational/Attitudinal	Behavioral	Health
■ Understands that healthy eating behaviors and regular physical activity are crucial to growth, development, and health ■ Understands the importance of eating a variety of healthy foods and how to increase food variety ■ Understands the importance of a healthy diet consisting of 3 meals per day and snacks as needed ■ Understands the physical, emotional, and social benefits of regular physical activity and how to increase physical activity level ■ Understands that people come in unique body sizes and shapes, within a range of healthy body weights ■ Understands safe ways to achieve and maintain a healthy body weight, and recognizes the dangers of unsafe weight-loss and weight-gain methods	■ Consumes a variety of healthy foods ■ Makes healthy food choices at and away from home ■ Seldom skips meals and does not practice restrictive eating or eating disorder behaviors ■ Participates in a moderate amount of physical activity on most, if not all, days of the week	■ Maintains optimal nutrition to promote growth and development ■ Achieves nutritional and physical well-being, without signs of iron-deficiency anemia, undernutrition, obesity, eating disorders, dental caries, or other nutrition-related problems ■ Achieves and maintains a healthy body weight and positive body image

(continued)

Table 6. Desired Outcomes for the Adolescent, and the Role of the Family (continued)

Family

Educational/Attitudinal	Behavioral	Health
■ Understands the nutrition needs of the growing adolescent ■ Understands physical changes that occur with growth and development ■ Understands the relationship between nutrition and short- and long-term health ■ Understands the importance of a healthy diet consisting of 3 meals per day and snacks as needed ■ Understands that people come in unique body sizes and shapes, within a range of healthy body weights ■ Understands the dangers of unsafe weight-loss methods, and knows safe ways to achieve and maintain a healthy weight	■ Provides a positive role model: practices healthy eating behaviors, participates in regular physical activity, and promotes a positive body image ■ Provides a variety of healthy foods at home, limiting the availability of high-fat and high-sugar foods ■ Eats meals together regularly to ensure optimal nutrition and to facilitate family communication ■ Provides opportunities for the adolescent to participate in meal planning and food preparation ■ Uses community nutrition programs and food resources if needed ■ Participates in regular physical activity with the adolescent	■ Provides developmentally appropriate, healthy foods and modifies them if necessary ■ Helps the adolescent achieve and maintain a healthy weight ■ Provides opportunities and safe places for the adolescent to participate in physical activity

References

1. Story M. 1992. Nutritional requirements during adolescence. In McAnarney ER, Kreipe RE, Orr DE, Comerci GD, eds., *Textbook of Adolescent Medicine.* Philadelphia, PA: WB Saunders, pp. 75–84.

2. Pollitt E, Mathews R. 1998. Breakfast and cognition: An integrative summary. *American Journal of Clinical Nutrition* 67(4):804S–813S.

3. Centers for Disease Control and Prevention. 1996. Guidelines for school health programs to promote lifelong eating. *Morbidity and Mortality Weekly Report* 45(RR-9):1–41.

4. Centers for Disease Control and Prevention. 1997. Guidelines for school and community programs to promote lifelong physical activity among young people. *Morbidity and Mortality Weekly Report* 46(RR-6):1–36.

5. Munoz KA, Krebs-Smith SM, Ballard-Barbash R, Cleveland LE. 1997. Food intakes of US children and adolescents compared with recommendations. *Pediatrics* 100(3):323–329.

6. Troiano RP, Flegal KM. 1998. Overweight children and adolescents: Description, epidemiology, and demographics. *Pediatrics* 101(Suppl. 1):497–504.

7. World Health Organization. 1995. Physical status: The use and interpretation of anthropometry. Report of a WHO expert committee. *World Health Organization Technical Report Series* 854:1–452.

8. Himes JH, Dietz WH. 1994. Guidelines for overweight in adolescent preventive services: Recommendations from an expert committee. *American Journal of Clinical Nutrition* 59:307–316.

9. Centers for Disease Control and Prevention, Epidemiology Program Office. 1998. *Recommendations to Prevent and Control Iron Deficiency in the United States.* Atlanta, GA: Centers for Disease Control and Prevention, Epidemiology Program Office.

10. American Dental Association. 1998. *ADA Guide to Dental Therapeutics.* Chicago, IL: ADA Publishing Co.

Suggested Reading

Green M, Palfrey JS, eds. 2000. *Bright Futures: Guidelines for Health Supervision of Infants, Children, and Adolescents* (2nd ed.). Arlington, VA: National Center for Education in Maternal and Child Health.

ADOLESCENCE • 11–21 YEARS

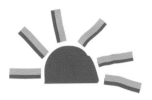

A Dancer's Dream

Katherine's mother is concerned that Katherine appears to be "chunky" and thinks that she will probably need to slim down if she is going to have a chance of making the team.

Katherine Gomez is a seventh-grade student attending middle school. She loves to dance and has been taking lessons since she was 5 years old. Katherine has dreamed of being on her school's dance team, and now, as a seventh-grader, she can try out for the team. Katherine's mother is concerned that Katherine appears to be "chunky" and thinks that she will probably need to slim down if she is going to have a chance of making the team. Mrs. Gomez asks their physician, Dr. Meyer, for a diet for Katherine.

Dr. Meyer measures Katherine's weight and height, and determines her body mass index (BMI). He assures Katherine and Mrs. Gomez that Katherine's weight and height are well proportioned and within the normal range for her age. Dr. Meyer explains that Katherine's body is preparing for the adolescent growth spurt by laying down extra fat and that it could be harmful to Katherine's health to restrict her calorie intake. He also asks Katherine about her eating behaviors and determines that they are appropriate for her age. Dr. Meyer advises Katherine to eat three meals a day and to eat nutritious snacks when she is hungry. He suggests that she try to eat a wide variety of foods and to choose fruits, vegetables, and low-fat dairy foods as snacks rather than chips, candy, and soft drinks.

Dr. Meyer realizes that Katherine and her mother need additional information and guidance on anticipated physical changes and nutrition needs during adolescence. The physician refers Mrs. Gomez and her daughter to a dietitian for follow-up. He also makes a note in Katherine's chart to evaluate her height, weight, and food intake during her next visit.

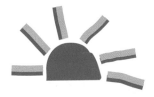

Helping an Active Adolescent Manage Diabetes

Charlie Davis is an active 14-year-old who loves to play basketball. One afternoon, he rushes home from school to tell his parents that he wants to try out for the basketball team. The coach has seen Charlie play basketball with his classmates and thinks that he could become a good player. Mr. and Mrs. Davis are happy for their son, but also concerned. Charlie was diagnosed with diabetes 6 months ago. It took the family almost 2 months to learn how to balance his food intake and insulin dose to keep his blood glucose in a healthy range. If Charlie decides to play basketball, it could mean that the family would have to change its routine again.

Mr. and Mrs. Davis call their physician, Dr. Yamaguchi, for advice. They ask how risky it would be for Charlie to play on a basketball team and how it could affect his insulin levels. Dr. Yamaguchi assures Mr. and Mrs. Davis that many adolescents with diabetes are physically active. Dr. Yamaguchi suggests that Charlie and his parents come in for a visit if he makes the basketball team.

Charlie makes the team, and his parents reluctantly agree to let him play if he learns how to adjust his food intake and insulin dose. At the diabetes clinic, members of the health care team show Charlie and his parents how to monitor his blood glucose level to learn how physical activity will affect it, and how to treat a low-blood-glucose reaction (hypoglycemia). Charlie is taught to carry fast-acting carbohydrate snacks and glucose to consume if he becomes hypoglycemic. His eating schedule is altered to include a snack before and after each practice and game. Charlie also learns how to choose appropriate foods from fast-food and other restaurants when his team travels, and he is advised that post-exercise hypoglycemia may occur 4 to 10 hours after unusually intense or long workouts. The health care team suggests that Charlie and his parents talk with the coach about his special health needs, and that the coach be taught how to identify and treat hypoglycemia. The health care team asks Charlie to schedule a follow-up visit.

During the follow-up visit, Charlie reports that he is doing well. It took a couple of weeks for him to learn what types of pregame snacks he needs to keep his blood glucose levels from dropping too low, but he has not had a low-blood-glucose reaction since the second week of practice. He is excited to share that he has been picked as a starting player for the team.

FREQUENTLY ASKED QUESTIONS ABOUT NUTRITION IN ADOLESCENCE

■ **How can I encourage my teenager to eat healthy foods?**

Serve new foods and regional and ethnic foods.

Involve the family in shopping, cooking, and trying new foods.

Be a positive role model—practice healthy eating behaviors yourself.

Don't fight over food with your teenager.

Keep a variety of healthy foods in the house. Limit the availability of high-fat and high-sugar foods.

■ **How can our family eat healthy meals together when our schedules are so busy?**

Try eating different meals together (for example, sometimes breakfast and other times lunch or dinner).

Buy healthy ready-to-eat meals from the store or healthy take-out foods from a restaurant.

Have family members share the cooking. Use food preparation and cooking as a family activity.

When your family eats together, use the time to socialize. Avoid distractions. Turn the television off, and don't answer the telephone.

■ **How can I encourage my teenager to eat breakfast?**

Provide foods that are fast and easy to prepare (for example, bagels, fruit, or yogurt).

Serve foods other than the usual breakfast foods (for example, sandwiches, baked potatoes, and leftovers such as chicken or pasta).

Help your teenager get organized so that she has time to eat in the morning.

Prepare breakfast the night before.

If your teenager is in a hurry, suggest that she take some food (for example, fresh fruits or trail mix) to eat on the bus or at school.

If your teenager is not hungry, offer a breakfast shake (for example, low-fat milk, fruit, and ice mixed in a blender).

Explain that skipping breakfast can lead to out-of-control hunger, which may cause overeating later. If your teenager is worried about gaining excess weight, offer low-fat foods.

■ **How can I get my teenager to eat more fruits and vegetables?**

Be a role model—eat more fruits and vegetables yourself.

Have your teenager take a piece of fruit to eat at school.

Keep juice in the refrigerator.

Keep a variety of fresh fruits and vegetables in the home.

Put a bowl of fruit on the kitchen table or counter.

Wash and cut up fruits and vegetables and keep them in a clear container (so they can be seen easily) in the refrigerator, along with low-fat dip or salsa.

Serve two or more vegetables with dinner (including at least one your teenager likes). Serve a salad with a choice of dressing.

Use plenty of vegetables in soups, sauces, and casseroles.

Plant a garden.

Offer a variety of fruits and vegetables at meals and snacks, but don't force your teenager to eat them.

■ **How can I help my teenager, who does not drink milk, get enough calcium?**

Use low-fat dairy foods, such as low-fat or skim milk, in recipes (for example, in puddings, milk-shakes, soups, casseroles, and cooked cereals).

Have low-fat dairy foods available for snacks (for example, cheese, yogurt, and frozen yogurt).

Offer unusual dairy foods, such as yogurt juice drinks and new flavors of low-fat yogurt.

Serve other calcium-rich foods such as tofu (if processed with calcium sulfate) and greens such as broccoli and turnip greens.

Serve calcium-fortified foods (for example, orange juice or cereal).

If your adolescent is lactose intolerant, suggest the following: small, frequent portions of milk and other dairy foods; milk with a snack or meal; yogurt or reduced-lactose milk; aged hard cheeses (for example, Cheddar, Colby, Swiss, and Parmesan) that are low in lactose; or lactase tablets or drops.

If these strategies don't work, consider giving your teenager a calcium supplement.

■ **How can I teach my teenager to make healthy food choices away from home?**

Encourage your teenager to make healthy food choices when buying food at school, stores, and restaurants, and from vending machines.

Review school and restaurant menus with your teenager and discuss healthy food choices. Identify items on these menus that are low in fat and calories.

Encourage your teenager to eat salads, low-calorie dressings, and broiled or baked meats.

Encourage your teenager to avoid eating fried foods or to reduce the serving size (for example, splitting an order of French fries with a friend).

Teach your teenager to be assertive and to request food modifications (for example, asking the server to "hold the mayonnaise").

■ **My teenager snacks on high-fat and high-sugar foods. What should I do?**

Limit the availability of high-fat and high-sugar foods at home (for example, chips, candy, and soft drinks).

Keep a variety of easy-to-prepare and healthy foods on hand.

Stock up on healthy snack foods (for example, pretzels, baked chips, popcorn, juice, fruits, vegetables, low-fat granola bars, and yogurt).

Wash and cut up vegetables and keep them in a clear container (so they can be seen easily) in the refrigerator, along with low-fat dip or salsa.

Put a bowl of fruit on the kitchen table or counter.

Encourage your teenager to make healthy food choices when buying food at school, stores, and restaurants, and from vending machines.

■ **My teenager has become a vegetarian. Should I be concerned?**

With careful planning, a vegetarian lifestyle can be healthy and meet the needs of a growing teenager.

A vegetarian diet that includes dairy foods and eggs usually provides adequate nutrients; however, your teenager may need to take an iron supplement.

Vegans are strict vegetarians who don't eat any animal products, including dairy foods, eggs, and fish. They may need additional calcium, vitamin B_{12}, and vitamin D, which can be provided by fortified foods and supplements.

Instead of always preparing separate vegetarian meals for your teenager, occasionally fix vegetarian meals for the whole family.

Ask a dietitian or nutritionist to help you plan healthy meals.

■ What should I do if my teenager seems overweight?

If your teenager is growing, eats healthy foods, and is physically active, you do not need to worry about whether he is overweight.

Let your teenager know that people come in unique sizes and shapes and that he is loved regardless of size and shape. Never criticize the teenager's size or shape.

If others comment about the size or shape of your teenager, redirect their comments to your teenager's other attributes.

Be a positive role model—practice healthy eating behaviors and participate in regular physical activity yourself.

Focus on gradually changing the entire family's eating behaviors and physical activity practices instead of singling out the overweight teenager.

Plan family activities that everyone enjoys (for example, hiking, biking, or swimming).

Limit to 1 to 2 hours per day the amount of time your teenager watches TV and videotapes and plays computer games.

Serve scheduled meals and snacks.

Reduce the amount of high-fat and high-sugar foods in your family's meals and snacks.

Do not forbid sweets and desserts. Serve them in moderation.

Encourage your teenager to avoiding dieting to lose weight, unless a health professional recommends a diet for medical reasons and supervises it.

■ How can I help my teenager like her body?

Teenagers are very sensitive about comments related to their appearance. Do not criticize your teenager about her size or shape.

Be a positive role model—don't criticize your own size or shape or that of others.

Focus on traits other than appearance when talking to your teenager.

Discuss how the media affects your teenager's body image.

■ How can I help my underweight teenager gain weight?

Limit the quantity of beverages your teenager drinks between meals if his appetite is being affected.

Encourage your teenager to eat a midmorning snack at school, if possible, and an after-school snack. Limit snacks close to mealtimes if snacking is affecting his appetite.

Have your teenager help with meal planning and food preparation.

Continue to offer foods even if your teenager has refused to eat them before. Your teenager is more likely to accept these foods after they have been offered several times.

■ **How can I encourage my teenager to be more physically active?**

Encourage active, spur-of-the-moment physical activity.

Limit to 1 to 2 hours per day the time your teenager spends watching television and video-tapes and playing computer games.

For every hour your teenager reads, watches tele-vision and videotapes, or plays computer games, encourage her to take a 10-minute physical activity break.

Involve your teenager in family chores (for example, raking leaves or walking the dog).

Plan at least one special physical activity (for example, taking a hike or riding a bike) each week.

Incorporate physical activities with your teenager into your daily life (for example, by using the stairs instead of taking an elevator or escalator, and by walking or riding a bike instead of driving a car).

Be a positive role model—participate in physical activity yourself.

Participate in physical activity together (for example, biking, dancing, or skating).

Encourage your teenager to enroll in planned physical activities (for example, swimming, mar-tial arts, gymnastics, or dancing).

Work with community leaders to ensure that your teenager has safe places for participating in physical activity (for example, walking and bik-ing paths, playgrounds, parks, and community centers).

■ **What are common symptoms of eating disorders?**

Common symptoms of anorexia nervosa are as follows:

Excessive weight loss in a short period of time

Continuation of dieting although thin

Dissatisfaction with appearance; belief that body is fat, even though severely thin

Loss of menstrual period

Unusual interest in certain foods and development of unusual eating rituals

Eating in secret

Obsession with exercise

Depression

Common symptoms of bulimia nervosa are as follows:

Loss of menstrual period

Unusual interest in certain foods and development of unusual eating rituals

Eating in secret

Obsession with exercise

Depression

Binge-eating

Binge-eating with no noticeable weight gain

Vomiting or laxative use

Disappearance into bathroom for long periods of time (e.g., to induce vomiting)

Alcohol or drug abuse

Resources for Health Professionals and Families

Clark N. 1996. *Nancy Clark's Sports Nutrition Guidebook* (2nd ed.). Champaign, IL: Human Kinetics.

Dietz WH, Stern L, eds. 1999. *Guide to Your Child's Nutrition: Making Peace at the Table and Building Healthy Eating Habits for Life.* Elk Grove Village, IL: American Academy of Pediatrics.

National Institutes of Health, National Institute of Diabetes and Digestive and Kidney Diseases. 1997. *Helping Your Overweight Child.* Bethesda, MD: National Institutes of Health, National Institute of Diabetes and Digestive and Kidney Diseases.

National Institutes of Health, National Institute of Mental Health. 1993. *Eating Disorders.* Bethesda, MD: National al Institutes of Health, National Institute of Mental Health.

Nissenberg SK, Bogle ML, Wright AC. 1995. *Quick Meals for Healthy Kids and Busy Parents.* New York, NY: John Wiley and Sons.

Rickert VI, ed. 1996. *Adolescent Nutrition: Assessment and Management.* New York, NY: Chapman and Hall.

Storlie J. 1997. *Snacking Habits for Healthy Living.* Minneapolis, MN: Chronimed Publishing.

Tamborlane WV, Weiswasser JZ, Held NA, Fung T. 1997. *The Yale Guide to Children's Nutrition.* New Haven, CT: Yale University Press.

U.S. Department of Agriculture, Food and Consumer Service. 1997. *Fun Tips: Using the Dietary Guidelines at Home.* Alexandria, VA: U.S. Department of Agriculture, Food and Consumer Service. In USDA's Team Nutrition [Web site]. Cited August 13, 1999; available at http://151.121.3.25/teanut/Resources/funtips.html or by written request to USDA's Team Nutrition, 3101 Park Center Drive, Room 1010, Alexandria, VA 22302.

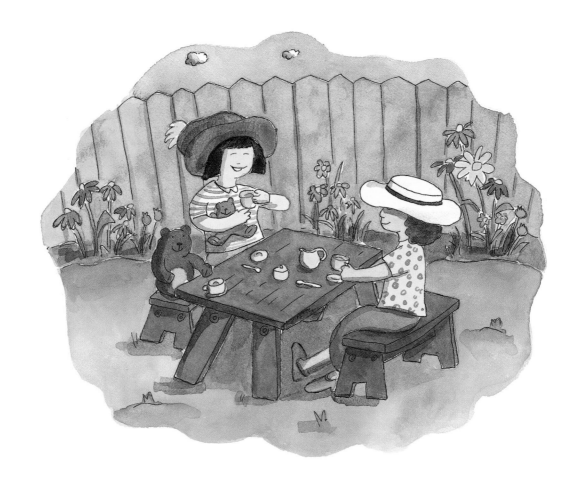

Nutrition
Issues and Concerns

BREASTFEEDING

In the United States, 60 percent of mothers breastfeed their infants for a brief period, with fewer than 25 percent of infants receiving any breastmilk by 6 months of age. The *Healthy People 2010* objectives for breastfeeding are to achieve, among women in the United States, levels of 75 percent who initiate breastfeeding and of 50 percent who maintain breastfeeding for at least 6 months.[1] To achieve these objectives, it is essential that health professionals and parents recognize the enormous benefits of breastfeeding and breastmilk and understand how to effectively manage lactation.

Most infants born in the United States in the 20th century have not been breastfed. Cow's milk preparations and other infant formulas were usually adopted as the major source of nutrition during the first year of life. However, research during the past 20 years has repeatedly demonstrated the importance of breastmilk for infants. This recognition of the health, nutritional, immunological, psychological, and societal advantages of breastmilk over all substitutes has led to a gradual increase in breastfeeding, especially during the first 2 to 4 months of life. Recently, additional health benefits from breastfeeding—as well as economic and environmental advantages—for mothers have been defined.[2,3]

The Benefits of Breastfeeding

Breastfeeding provides infants with significant protection against a variety of infectious diseases, particularly in areas of the world with poor sanitation and contaminated water and food supplies. Epidemiological studies in the United States and other developed countries have shown that, compared with formula-fed infants, breastfed infants have fewer and less severe bacterial and viral diseases, including meningitis, gastroenteritis, otitis media, pneumonia, botulism, urinary tract infections, and necrotizing enterocolitis.[2,3]

There are a number of studies demonstrating that breastfeeding also helps prevent some chronic diseases, including type 1 diabetes mellitus, Crohn's disease, ulcerative colitis, lymphoma, and asthma and other allergic diseases.[2,3] Some of the preventive effects of breastfeeding (including those preventing otitis media and asthma) continue well

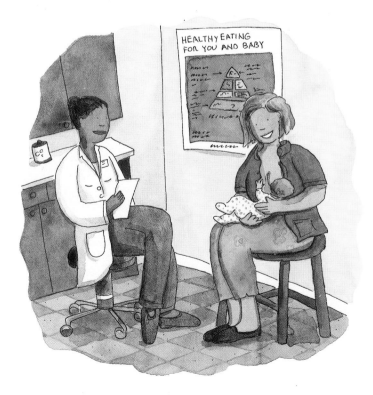

beyond the period of breastfeeding, suggesting that breastfeeding enhances long-term immunological response.[4] Moreover, growth patterns observed in the first year of life suggest that breastfeeding may help prevent obesity. Multiple studies have demonstrated an association between breastfeeding and improved cognitive behavior, including higher IQs and improved school performance through adolescence.

In the days after delivery, the mother's lactation reduces postpartum bleeding and the size of the uterus (an effect of oxytocin). The absence of menstruation during lactation reduces iron loss and delays the resumption of ovulation. Consequently, the time between pregnancies is increased, the risk of prematurity in later pregnancies is reduced, and adverse outcomes for the pregnancy or the infant are reduced. In proportion to the total duration of lactation, women who breastfeed have lower rates of ovarian cancer, premenopausal breast cancer, hip fractures, and osteoporosis.[2,3]

In the United States, hospitalizations, medical office visits, and pharmaceutical use are significantly reduced for breastfed infants, cutting health care costs by an average of $200 per breastfed infant compared with formula-fed infants.[5] Improved infant health reduces the loss of income due to parents' absence from work to care for the infant. Breastfeeding also eliminates or reduces the cost of purchasing infant formula, which has been estimated to range from $750 to $1,500 for the first year of life. Breast-pump rental and lactation consultation services may reduce some of these savings, but the net economic benefit is significant.

The Composition of Breastmilk

Human milk is radically different from cow's milk and even from prepared infant formula, despite attempts to modify formulas to make them similar to breastmilk. Breastmilk is extremely low in protein (about 0.9 g/100 mL) compared with raw cow's milk, which has nearly four times the concentration of protein.[6] Infant formulas are diluted to provide a low protein concentration that is comparable to human milk, but the protein structure (which is more difficult for the young infant to absorb) remains the same as that of cow's milk. In some formulas, the ratio of whey to casein is altered to make it comparable to breastmilk, in which whey is dominant. Because breastmilk's concentration of protein is very low, infants need to breastfeed frequently. Human milk proteins contain antibodies (known as secretory IgA) that are structured specifically to resist digestion.

The fats in breastmilk are very different from those in infant formulas and are absorbed better than those from animal or vegetable sources. Breastmilk also contains hundreds of micronutrients, including free amino acids, essential fatty acids, minerals, growth factors, cytokines, and other chemical agents that contribute to virtually every aspect of infant growth and development. Many of these components serve as both nutrients and bioactive agents to enhance the infant's development.

Breastmilk's composition varies during the course of breastfeeding. Colostrum, the initial milk, is higher in protein and lower in fat and lactose concentrations than mature milk.[6] Throughout the course of lactation, secretory IgA concentration gradually declines, allowing the infant's own immune system to develop and lose its dependency on the mother's sources. Because the mother and infant share the same environment, the mother develops and secretes specific antibodies to the viruses and bacteria to which the infant is exposed. This response is rapid, requiring only a few days. These dynamic changes in the composition of breastmilk show how well it adapts to meet the needs of the infant. Furthermore, breastmilk contains everything that the healthy, full-term infant requires for about the first 6 months of life, including water, vitamins, and minerals. (Some infants may require vitamin D or iron supplements.[2])

Initiating Breastfeeding

Breastfeeding is established most successfully when it is begun during the first hour after birth. The infant and mother should remain together throughout the recovery and postpartum period, with no interruptions in the "rooming-in." The mother should be encouraged to put her infant to the breast at the earliest signs of hunger (e.g., mouthing motions, hand-to-mouth movements, wide-eyed eagerness, cooing).[2] Crying is a late sign of hunger that often interferes with good breastfeeding; the crying infant usually requires calming before breastfeeding can begin. Positioning and latching-on require some initial experimentation. A good "let-down" sensation (tingling in the breast) accompanied by brief cramping pain in the uterus (from the release of oxytocin by the pituitary gland) are signs of a good latch-on. Counseling by a lactation expert can often identify problems in positioning and latching-on that can be easily corrected before unnecessary pain and nipple injury occur.

Mothers should breastfeed at least 8 to 12 times every 24 hours during the early weeks of lactation, and the infant should be allowed to feed at both breasts for as long as desired during each feeding session. Frequent breastfeeding and complete emptying of both breasts will help prevent engorgement. The hind milk—the portion that comes out toward the end of emptying a breast—contains much more fat, which provides essential calories and signals the infant to end feeding on that breast.[4] Water and formula supplementation are not needed and should be discouraged, because they will interfere with the development of good breastfeeding patterns. Water supplementation also increases the likelihood that the infant will not consume as many calories and subsequently develop jaundice and severe hyperbilirubinemia. The use of pacifiers should also be discouraged during the early weeks of life, when they may complicate breastfeeding initiation and cause premature weaning.[2]

The adequacy of the infant's milk intake can be evaluated by the mother and health professionals by observing whether the infant has five or more wet diapers and three or four stools per day by 5 to 7 days of age. A trained observer should evaluate the breastfeeding position, latch-on, and sucking and swallowing during the first few days. Within 2 to 3 days after discharge from the hospital, the mother and infant should be seen by a physician or other health professional trained in lactation management to evaluate the breastfeeding.[2] At this time, infants should be weighed; if they have lost more than 7 percent of their birthweight, the mother's breastfeeding practices should be evaluated and corrected if necessary to increase milk production and feeding. Nipple pain and cracking, breast engorgement, and all other problems should also be addressed to ensure that breastfeeding is successful. If problems are not evaluated and corrected at this point, breastfeeding may be stopped too early.

Mothers should be able to obtain counseling from a lactation expert by phone and in person when needed. Home visits by lactation consultants, nurses, nutritionists, and/or physicians trained in breastfeeding can be very helpful in evaluating and correcting breastfeeding problems. Peer support groups (e.g., La Leche League) are also helpful throughout infancy, especially when the mother is initiating breastfeeding and adapting to her new infant.

The Mother's Diet

During the early weeks of breastfeeding, the mother does not need to eat more food than she would have eaten before pregnancy. Fat stores provide adequate energy sources for milk production. Encourage the mother to drink extra fluids (especially milk, juice, and water) to keep from getting thirsty. Breastfeeding accelerates the mother's return to her prepregnancy weight and shape. However, after about 6 weeks, lactating mothers need to eat more to satisfy their hunger. An increase of about 600 to 800 calories and about a quart of water per day is usually sufficient. A well-balanced diet is adequate, and no special foods or nutrient groups are required.

While most foods (including spicy and exotic ones) eaten by the mother are well tolerated by breastfeeding infants, occasionally the infant may have symptoms that suggest allergy or intolerance. For example, cow's milk protein enters the breastmilk and has been shown to result in sensitization and allergic symptoms in about 8 percent of breast-fed infants. In these cases, the mother may need to

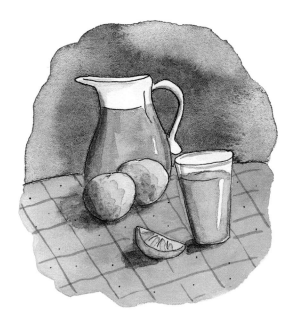

eliminate known or suspected allergenic foods from her diet. The mother's caffeine intake should be eliminated or reduced, because it may lead to prolonged waking periods or agitation in the infant. Alcohol intake during lactation should also be eliminated or at least restricted to only an occasional single drink, because alcohol is readily transferred into breastmilk and can intoxicate the infant.

Continuing Breastfeeding

Breastmilk provides sufficient nutrition for about the first 6 months of life and should be encouraged. Iron-fortified infant cereal, which provides additional energy and iron, is a good choice for the first supplemental food given to infants. Healthy infants usually require little or no supplemental water (except in hot weather). Water is not needed during the first 6 months and should be offered thereafter only when conditions are extremely warm or when the infant has lost an excessive amount of water. Breastfeeding should be continued for at least the first year of life and into the second year and beyond for as long as both the mother and infant or child desire it. The benefits of breastfeeding for both mother and infant or child continue for as long as breastfeeding is practiced. However, after 6 months of age, infants living in areas where the water supply is severely deficient in fluoride (less than 0.3 ppm) should receive oral fluoride supplements.[2]

Some mothers may wish to breastfeed and formula-feed their infants, perhaps because they have returned to work or school outside of the home. Mixed feeding should be discouraged during the early weeks of breastfeeding because it often interferes with the establishment of a good breastmilk supply and may lead to premature weaning from the breast.[7] To maintain her milk supply and avoid engorgement, the mother needs to breastfeed or pump her breasts frequently and regularly every day. Some mothers may be able to adapt their breastfeeding schedule after a few months so that they can go 6 to 8 hours during the day without pumping and then breastfeed the infant frequently in the evening and at night.

For mothers returning to work or school, breastfeeding can be effectively maintained by pumping about every 4 hours and storing the expressed breastmilk in a cooled container (e.g., an insulated bag with ice packs, a prefrozen insulated vacuum bottle). This milk can then be stored in the refrigerator for up to 48 hours, for feeding to the infant the following day by bottle or cup, or it can be frozen for 3 to 6 months if stored at 0°F in the back of the freezer. Breastmilk should never be stored in the door of a freezer or refrigerator. Sterile or well-cleaned hard plastic or glass containers are suitable for storing breastmilk. Frozen breastmilk should be thawed slowly either at room tempera-

ture, in the refrigerator, or in a warm-water bath. Breastmilk should never be warmed in a microwave oven since it can easily overheat, burning the infant and destroying the beneficial qualities of the milk.

Mothers who plan to go back to work or school should talk with their employer or school about the need for a private place and time to pump. Some employers purchase high-grade electric breast pumps for employees' use and allow sufficient time to use them. These arrangements benefit an organization financially because employees' absences to care for their infants or children, as well as health insurance costs, may be reduced, and employee satisfaction and retention will improve.

Weaning should occur naturally and gradually when the mother and infant are ready, although preferably not before the infant's first birthday.[2,7] The most comfortable way to wean is for mothers to gradually reduce the frequency of breastfeeding and replace breastmilk with other foods and milks over a period of several weeks. For infants, only iron-fortified infant formula is appropriate as a substitute for breastmilk.[2]

Contraindications to Breastfeeding

While breastmilk is the best food for almost every infant, breastfeeding and breastmilk in some cases may be contraindicated, either temporarily or permanently.[2,3]

The strongest contraindication is when the infant has an inherited metabolic disorder such as galactosemia, in which the infant is unable to metabolize the galactose portion of the milk sugar called lactose. Lactose elimination must then be instituted for the infant, and the infant should not be breastfed. Infants with phenylketonuria may continue to receive breastmilk (because of its low protein concentration) if they are monitored carefully for blood phenylalanine levels. There are other inherited disorders that contraindicate breastfeeding, but they are rare.

Although HIV infection and untreated active pulmonary tuberculosis are contraindications to breastfeeding in the United States and other developed countries, most maternal infections do not contraindicate breastfeeding.[2,3] Maternal hepatitis A, B, and C are not transmitted in breastmilk. Cytomegalovirus infection via breastmilk may be a risk to premature infants, but it is not a risk to full-term infants. A mother who develops a fever or other signs of infection while breastfeeding (whether from a viral or bacterial infection) has already exposed her infant to the infection and should be encouraged to continue breastfeeding the infant or to express breastmilk; the breastmilk will provide specific antibodies and other nonspecific anti-infectious agents to protect the infant. In fact, removing the infant from breastfeeding may increase the infant's risk of developing the infection. Mastitis does not harm the infant, and the continuation of breastfeeding is essential to hasten the mother's recovery. Breastfeeding may even be continued with breast abscesses, as long as the incision and surgical drainage tube are far enough away from the areola that they are not involved in feeding.

Breastfeeding mothers can take most drugs, whether prescription or over-the-counter. Radioactive isotopes, certain antimetabolites, and a few antibiotics and antipsychosis drugs are contraindicated during breastfeeding. Every effort should be made to substitute safe drugs and/or maintain lacta-tion by pumping while the drugs are being administered. Excellent references are available to identify which drugs are safe and which are not.[8,9] Oral contraceptives of low-dose progesterone are safe and compatible with breastfeeding, but estrogen-containing agents should be avoided because they may inhibit milk production.

Summary

Breastmilk is a valuable, readily available resource with extensive short- and long-term benefits for both mother and infant. It is essential that health professionals understand the benefits and management of breastfeeding and that this topic be included in their education and training.[10] Health professionals can thus help ensure the improved health and development of almost all infants, children, and adolescents.

References

1. U.S. Department of Health and Human Services. 2000. *Healthy People 2010: National Health Promotion and Disease Prevention Objectives*. Washington, DC: U.S. Department of Health and Human Services.

2. American Academy of Pediatrics, Work Group on Breastfeeding. 1997. Breastfeeding and the use of human milk [policy statement no. RE9729]. *Pediatrics* 100(6):1035–1039.

3. Lawrence RA. 1997. *A Review of the Medical Benefits and Contraindications to Breastfeeding in the United States*. Arlington, VA: National Center for Education in Maternal and Child Health.

4. Horwood LJ, Fergusson DM. 1998. Breastfeeding and later cognitive and academic outcomes. *Pediatrics* 101(1):e9.

5. Montgomery DL, Splett PL. 1997. Economic benefit of breast-feeding in infants enrolled in WIC. *Journal of The American Dietetic Association* 97(4):379–385.

6. Lawrence RA. 1999. *Breastfeeding: A Guide for the Medical Profession* (5th ed.). St. Louis, MO: Mosby-Year Book.

7. La Leche League International. 1997. *The Womanly Art of Breastfeeding* (6th ed.). Schaumburg, IL: La Leche League International.

8. Briggs GG, Freeman RK, Yaffe SJ. 1998. *Drugs in Pregnancy and Lactation* (5th ed.). Baltimore, MD: Williams and Wilkins.

9. Hale TW. 1999. *Medications and Mothers' Milk* (8th ed.). Amarillo, TX: Pharmasoft Medical Publishing.

10. Gartner LM, Newton ER. 1998. Breastfeeding: Role of the obstetrician. *ACOG Clinical Review* 3:1–15.

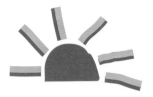

Supporting an Adolescent Mother's Decision to Breastfeed

Denise Booker, a 17-year-old high-school junior who is single and pregnant, can't decide how to feed her baby. She is enrolled in WIC (Special Supplemental Nutrition Program for Women, Infants and Children) and has attended prenatal classes. All of the health professionals have emphasized the benefits of breastfeeding, pointing out the complete nutrient content of breastmilk, the lower risk of infection for babies, and the convenience of not having to sterilize bottles and prepare infant formula. Denise has also learned that she could complete her senior year at a high school that provides child care and would allow her to breastfeed her baby during school hours. She has become convinced that breastfeeding offers many advantages to her and her baby.

Denise's mother and the baby's father are trying to discourage Denise from breastfeeding. Both believe that breastfeeding will "tie her down" to the baby and will interfere with their ability to care for the baby. Denise's mother bottlefed all of her children and she thinks it is

Denise has also learned that she could complete her senior year at a high school that provides child care and would allow her to breastfeed her baby during school hours.

unnecessary to have to pump breastmilk when infant formula is widely available. She has also expressed uneasiness about handling expressed breastmilk when she is caring for her grandchild.

Denise discusses her dilemma with the WIC nutritionist, Mariana Rivera. They set up a meeting at which Denise, her mother, and her boyfriend talk openly about the issue of breastfeeding vs. bottlefeeding. The nutritionist plays a videotape that demonstrates the techniques for breastfeeding

and for feeding expressed breastmilk. After a thorough discussion, they all agree to support Denise's desire to breastfeed her baby.

After the baby is born, a lactation consultant visits Denise in the hospital. She helps Denise position the baby for breastfeeding and explains the baby's natural reflex to search for the nipple and begin suckling. The consultant shows Denise how to tell if the baby is properly latched on to the breast and swallowing milk. Before Denise and her baby leave the hospital, the lactation consultant gives Denise some pamphlets and other educational materials on breastfeeding as well as a listing of local resources. The consultant tells Denise that she will call in a few days to find out how things are going and to answer any questions.

NUTRITION AND SPORTS

I n competitive sports, strength training, and fitness activities, nutrition plays an important role in the promotion of healthy eating and weight management strategies. These strategies enhance performance and endurance while ensuring optimal growth, health, and physical and emotional development.

Significance

Children and adolescents are encouraged to engage in regular physical activity to promote life-long fitness. The benefits of appropriate physical activity include the following:

- Decreased risk of cardiovascular and other chronic diseases

- Maintenance of healthy body weight

- Promotion of an appropriate level of body fat

- Increased cardiopulmonary health

- Increased muscular strength, flexibility, and endurance

- Decreased anxiety, stress, and depression

- Enhanced self-esteem

Young athletes are particularly vulnerable to misinformation about nutrition and to claims about unsafe practices that promise enhanced performance. Pressure to achieve that "competitive edge" encourages athletes to experiment with ergogenic aids (e.g., instant protein beverages; weight-gain powders; amino acid, herbal, vitamin, and mineral supplements). Many ergogenic aids offer no benefits, and some are actually harmful.

Inappropriate use of dietary supplements, unsafe weight-control methods, and unhealthy eating practices can adversely affect strength and endurance, jeopardize health, and negate the benefits of training. Research continues to support recommendations to improve performance through a combination of safe training and healthy eating practices.

Nutritional Adequacy

Children and adolescents who are physically active and those who compete in sports can achieve an adequate, balanced intake of nutrients by following the Dietary Guidelines for Americans.[1] The nutrient needs of young athletes are similar to those of noncompeting children and adolescents, with the exception of energy, water, and, in some cases, protein.[2]

Energy

Physical activity increases the body's need for energy in relation to the type, frequency, intensity, and duration of the activity. Most young athletes need approximately 500 to 1,500 additional calories per day; adequacy of growth, appropriate body weight status, and appetite indicate whether the energy intake is sufficient.

Carbohydrates

Carbohydrates are the preferred source of energy for exercising the muscles. Inadequate carbohydrate intake may be associated with fatigue and decreased performance. For those who are physically active or competing, a higher proportion of car-

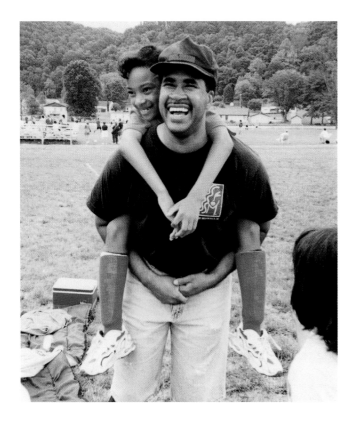

bohydrates (especially complex carbohydrates such as grains, corn, and potatoes) is recommended, in addition to fruits, vegetables, low-fat dairy products, and moderate sugar intake.[3] For highly trained athletes competing at the national or international level, the recommended carbohydrate intake is 60 to 70 percent of total calories consumed; for young athletes, 55 to 65 percent is probably more realistic.

Protein

The protein requirements of most young athletes can be met by consuming approximately 1 g protein per kg body weight per day. Athletes engaging in intense endurance sports or strength training may require 1.5 to 2 g protein per kg body weight per day;[3] however, most children and adolescents consume 1.5 to 3 times their RDA for pro-

tein, so it is likely that protein needs can be met by eating a variety of nutritious foods (unless an athlete is restricting food intake).

Higher consumption of proteins and the use of protein or amino acid supplements (misleadingly promoted as "safe" alternatives to steroids) are not beneficial and may cause dehydration, renal stress, increased urinary excretion of calcium, and excessive caloric intake and fat storage. Athletes who eat increased amounts of protein or take amino acid supplements may tend to view these as substitutes for other foods, and thus neglect important nutrients.

Vitamins and Minerals

A balanced variety of foods that meet the body's energy needs also meet the requirement for sufficient vitamins and minerals. Adequate amounts of iron should be consumed to prevent iron-deficiency anemia, especially in menstruating females. If the athlete does not consume sufficient quantities of dairy products, a calcium supplement should be added.[4] Children and adolescents who perform strenuous activity may have a slightly increased need for zinc, but adequate zinc intake usually can be achieved by eating meats and whole grains.

Pregame and Postgame Meals

Consuming a light meal high in complex carbohydrates (e.g., rice, pasta, bread) and ample caffeine-free beverages (e.g., fruit juice, water) is recommended 3 to 4 hours before an event to prevent hunger, provide energy, ensure gastric emptying, and prevent respiratory and cardiac stress. During physical activities involving several events, energy can be obtained by consuming sports drinks or unsweetened fruit juice diluted to one-half strength with water up to 1 hour before physical activity. If events are 1 to 3 hours apart, carbohydrate snacks (e.g., cereal bars, sports bars, crackers, fruit) or liquid meals are recommended. After exercise, it is important to replace muscle and liver glycogen stores by consuming carbohydrates within 2 hours. Drinking beverages containing carbohydrates should be encouraged if foods are not well tolerated or not available within 2 hours after physical activity.

Fluids and Electrolytes

Adequate fluid intake and prevention of dehydration are critical for effective energy metabolism, performance, and body cooling. The risk of dehydration becomes greater with increased heat, humidity, intensity or duration of exercise, body surface area, and sweating. Children are at greater risk for dehydration and heat illness than adolescents or adults because children generate more heat, sweat less, take longer to acclimatize, and absorb more heat from the environment.

Inadequate fluid intake can result in dehydration and heat illness (see Table 7). To ensure adequate hydration in children and adolescents, note the following key principles:

- Adequate fluid intake must be ensured to prevent dehydration and serious problems, but thirst is not an adequate indication of the body's need for fluids.

- Drinking 16 oz of water 1 to 2 hours before the event is recommended, followed by 12 oz of water 15 minutes before the event and 4 to 8 oz of water every 15 to 20 minutes during the event.[3]

- During hot or humid weather, strenuous physical activity or events lasting more than 60 minutes,

muscle glycogen can be conserved and fatigue reduced by consuming drinks containing 4 to 8 percent carbohydrates (10–18 g carbohydrates per 8 oz). Examples include (1) unsweetened fruit juice diluted with an equal amount of water and (2) sports drinks.

- Cool water (40–50°F) is absorbed most quickly.

- Water can be more palatable for some children and adolescents if flavoring (e.g., lemon slices) is added.

- After physical activity, drinking 16 oz of fluid per pound of weight lost will restore water balance and allow optimal performance in subsequent exercise sessions.

- Undiluted fruit juice, carbonated or caffeine-containing beverages, and fruit punches should not be consumed immediately before or during physical activity because they may cause cramping or diarrhea.

- During hot weather, closely monitor children and adolescents who use exercise equipment (e.g., helmets, padding). These kinds of equipment can prevent sweat from evaporating, thus increasing body temperature.

Special Considerations

Anemia

Strenuous physical activity or intensive training may be associated with iron-deficiency anemia. Contributing factors include decreased iron absorption, marginal iron intake, hemodilution, increased destruction of erythrocytes in circulation, and foot strike hemolysis.[3] Iron-deficiency anemia is not a contraindication to continued training; however,

Table 7. Heat Illness: Signs, Symptoms, and Recommendations

	Signs and Symptoms	Health/Physical Status
Heat cramps	▪ Disabling muscular cramps ▪ Thirst ▪ Chills ▪ Rapid heart rate ▪ Normal body temperature ▪ Alertness ▪ Normal blood pressure ▪ Nausea	▪ Give child/adolescent 4–8 oz of cold water every 10–15 minutes ▪ Make sure child/adolescent avoids beverages that contain caffeine ▪ Move child/adolescent to shade ▪ Remove as much clothing and equipment as possible
Heat exhaustion	▪ Sweating ▪ Dizziness ▪ Headache ▪ Confusion ▪ Lightheadedness ▪ Clammy skin ▪ Flushed face ▪ Shallow breathing ▪ Nausea ▪ Body temperature of 100.4–104°F	▪ Give child/adolescent 16 oz of cold water for each pound of weight lost ▪ Move child/adolescent to a cool place ▪ Remove as much clothing and equipment as possible ▪ Cool child/adolescent (e.g., with ice baths, ice bags)
Heat stroke	▪ Shock ▪ Collapse ▪ Body temperature > 104°F ▪ Delirium ▪ Hallucinations ▪ Loss of consciousness ▪ Seizures ▪ Inability to walk	▪ Call for emergency medical treatment ▪ Cool child/adolescent (e.g., with ice packs, ice bags, immersion in ice water) ▪ Give intravenous fluids

Source: The information for this table was drawn from Maughan RJ, Shirreffs SM, eds.[5]

the anemic child's or adolescent's iron status should be evaluated by a health professional. (See the Iron-Deficiency Anemia chapter.)

Weight Status

Losing excess body fat is a long-term process involving healthy food choices as well as training. This process should be initiated several months before the start of the athletic season. Severe energy restriction and weight loss of more than 2 pounds per week can result in the loss of muscle mass and compromised growth and development. Weight maintenance and increased physical activity, rather than weight loss, are appropriate goals for growing athletes. Loss of body fat can be facilitated through physical activity (e.g., power walking, cycling) at 60 to 80 percent of maximum aerobic capacity (heart rate of 220 beats per minute minus age) for 45 to 60 minutes five to six times per week.

Rapid weight-loss techniques (e.g., severe food restriction, dehydration, purging) frequently practiced by athletes (e.g., wrestlers) are ineffective and dangerous. In addition to decreased muscle strength and endurance, side effects may include hypoglycemia, depletion of electrolytes and glycogen stores, nutrient deficiencies, risk of developing eating disorders, and compromised growth and development. Severe restriction can result in circulatory collapse and heat stroke. For example, wrestlers should be certified at their current weight unless they have excess body fat or are not experiencing growth; certification at a weight consistent with less than 7 percent body fat is contraindicated. Sufficient time should be allotted for gradual and appropriate weight loss.

Adolescents who wish to increase muscle mass should be advised to combine strength training with a balanced intake of healthy foods providing an additional 500 to 1,000 calories per day. This should result in a weight gain of 1 to 2 pounds per week. Foods chosen should be low in fat, cholesterol, and sugar, and high in complex carbohydrates.

Strength Training

Properly prescribed and supervised strength training as part of a total fitness program can improve body composition, increase muscular strength and endurance, reduce risk of injury, and enhance overall fitness and performance in sports and recreational activities. Strength training can increase muscle size in adolescents, but increased muscle mass beyond normal growth is not possible in children. To prevent injury of the long bones and back, children should not lift maximum or near-maximum weights. Weights that can be lifted for six repetitions or more are considered appropriate.[6]

Eating Disorders

Restricted food intake, binge eating, purging, and an unhealthy body image can occur among young athletes in all sports, but are more common in weight-related activities (e.g., wrestling, running) and in "appearance" sports (e.g., gymnastics, ballet, figure skating). Eating disorders may be associated with electrolyte imbalances, nutrient deficiencies, amenorrhea, and impaired growth and development. (See the Eating Disorders chapter.)

An issue of major concern in female athletes is the interrelationship between eating disorders, amenorrhea, and osteoporosis, which has been labeled the "Female Athlete Triad." Some female athletes may develop eating behaviors that can lead to weight loss, amenorrhea, and negative consequences for bone health (i.e., premature bone loss, decreased bone density, increased risk of stress fractures).[4] It is important to identify and treat this condition early, because bone disorders associated with anorexia may be irreversible despite estrogen replacement, calcium supplementation, and resumption of menstrual periods.

Creatine

Although creatine may promote increased muscle mass when combined with strength training, possible side effects include nausea and muscle cramps. There is insufficient information on the long-term risks of using creatine, and it is not recommended for young athletes.

Anabolic Steroids

Use of anabolic steroids by children and adolescents is dangerous and is banned by the National Collegiate Athletic Association and the International Olympic Committee. Although anabolic steroids may help build muscle, such steroids cause early closure of the epiphyseal plates, resulting in stunted growth. Children and adolescents who use such steroids are also at risk for sterility.

Screening and Assessment

The nutritional adequacy of typical eating practices as well as specialized training diets can be evaluated with the Food Guide Pyramid. To screen and assess children and adolescents for adequate nutrition, it is important to determine the following:

- Intake of calcium, iron, and zinc (from foods)

- Pregame and postgame eating practices

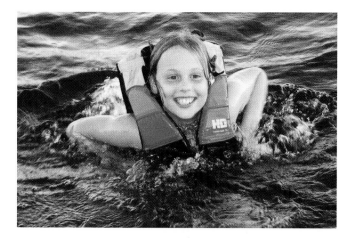

- Fluid intake before, during, and after competition

- Use of vitamin and mineral supplements

- Weight-control practices, including restrictive eating and binge-eating/purging activity

- Use of ergogenic aids (e.g., caffeine, steroids, amphetamines, creatine, chromium picolinate)

- Measurement of height, weight, and BMI annually to evaluate height-weight status and growth

- Measurement of body fat percentage (e.g., triceps skinfold) annually to distinguish excess body fat from excess body weight related to high muscularity

- Menstrual history

- Evaluation of type, frequency, intensity, and duration of physical activity to help determine energy needs

- For wrestlers, the determination of desired weight classification for competition, the sexual maturity rating, and training activities (urine specific gravity measurements may be indicated if dehydration before weight certification is suspected)

seling for oral health focused mainly on reducing carbohydrate intake.

However, over the past 30 years, the widespread availability of fluoride in drinking water and toothpaste has weakened the direct connection between carbohydrate intake and dental caries.[5] Today, nutrition screening and assessment in the context of oral health usually focus on (1) general risk assessment or (2) treating children and adolescents who present with significant oral disease. Evaluating children and adolescents with established oral disease (or with a systemic disease that is affecting the mouth) consists chiefly of taking a diet history (usually for 5 days, including a weekend) to assess carbohydrate intake (amount, frequency, and form) and general nutritional adequacy. Other specific nutrients may also be assessed, although the effect of deficiencies of trace elements and various minerals on oral health is unclear.

General risk assessment gives the dental professional the opportunity to tailor oral health supervision to the child's or adolescent's level of risk for specific diseases, conditions, and injuries. The assessment consists of (1) an interview to identify general, nutrition, and medical risk and protective factors for oral disease, and (2) an analysis of these factors to establish an oral health supervision plan, one that includes age-appropriate anticipatory guidance and recommendations on the type and frequency of visits needed. *Bright Futures in Practice: Oral Health* discusses general risk assessment and provides guidelines on risk factors for all children and adolescents and on those factors that are most common at a particular age.[6]

Nutrition Counseling

For children and adolescents with dental caries, nutrition counseling should examine the amount, frequency, consistency (e.g., stickiness), and timing of carbohydrate intake, particularly sugar. Children and adolescents with significant dental caries should be advised to cut back on the frequency of their carbohydrate intake, eat foods that are less sticky, eat snacks in moderation, and decrease their consumption of carbonated beverages, candy, and sports drinks.

Nutrition counseling for periodontal disease is not as straightforward as that for dental caries because the condition is more complex and takes years to emerge, but any nutrition counseling should stress eating a balanced diet that maintains the integrity of the gums and bones, supports immunity and healing, and, if possible, minimizes plaque accumulation. For other nutrition deficiencies and general medical conditions, nutrition counseling should be based on the specific condition, because any systemic therapy will most likely also benefit the mouth.

Some nutrition recommendations for oral health (e.g., good general nutrition, appropriate carbohydrate intake, adequate fluoride) can be given to all children and adolescents. Health professionals can use the following information to provide anticipatory guidance to parents, children, and adolescents.

Prenatal

Good maternal nutrition during pregnancy supports the formation of enamel of the infant's primary teeth. Extreme nutrition deficiencies in the mother can lead to malformed teeth in the infant, but the effect of borderline deficiencies is unknown. A woman's prenatal use of fluoride does not appear to give her fetus protection against future dental caries, but as a part of her general oral health maintenance, fluoride may reduce the level of caries-causing bacteria passed to the infant.[7]

Infancy and Early Childhood

When infants are 6 months old, the adequacy and method of their fluoride intake need to be addressed.[8] Systemic fluoride—that which is ingested through fluoridated water or fluoride supplements—becomes very important because of its long-term benefits. The level of fluoride in the public water supply and in the infant's formula, the parents' use of bottled water, the choice of fluoride supplement, and the absence of fluoride in breastmilk all need to be considered when determining how much fluoride the infant is ingesting.

Early childhood caries (baby bottle tooth decay), which is exacerbated by the excessive and inappropriate use of a bottle and transitional methods of feeding (e.g., tippy cup to cup), is another important concern. To reduce the risk of early childhood caries, infants and children should not be put to bed with a bottle or allowed to drink from a bottle at will during the day. Sucking on a bottle with any liquid (except water) for a prolonged period can contribute to tooth decay. Encouraging family members to practice good oral hygiene may help reduce the level of caries-causing bacteria that can be passed through the saliva by sharing food or utensils.

For young children in child care programs, nutrition-related oral health issues include access to carbohydrates and the fluoride levels in their vary-ing sources of drinking water. Nutrition safety concerns include fluoride toxicity (poisoning and fluorosis) and the potential for choking on foods (e.g., nuts, large pieces of meat).

Middle Childhood and Adolescence

Children's access to carbohydrate snacks, their snacking patterns, their increasing freedom in food choice outside the home, and their increasing energy needs are nutrition-related oral health issues. Children's consumption of their school's drinking water and bottled or processed water needs to be considered when evaluating the adequacy of their fluoride ingestion.

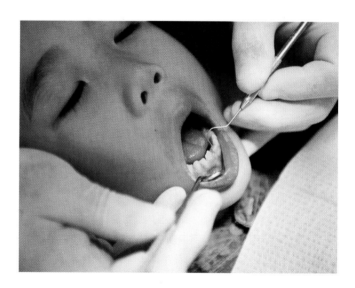

The type and frequency of snacks consumed by adolescents remain a concern. Dietary fads (e.g., sports drinks and high-citrus diets that decalcify teeth) can pose challenges to nutrition and oral health status. Bulimia nervosa can also erode teeth through a demineralization process similar to dental caries.[9] Adolescents' use of bottled and processed water may decrease their fluoride intake.

Children and Adolescents with Special Health Care Needs

Many diseases and conditions can affect the nutrition and oral health status of children and adolescents with special health care needs. Children and adolescents with any systemic illness that is managed through diet or that may damage their nutrition or oral health status should see a dentist regularly. Following are some of the implications that specific conditions and nutrition challenges have for oral health:

- Preterm and low-birthweight infants can exhibit oral and dental malformations.[10]

- Children and adolescents with special health care needs may require high-carbohydrate diets, which may in turn encourage dental caries. The frequency of carbohydrate feeding may also accelerate dental caries. The consistency of the foods (e.g., carbohydrate pastes) may encourage plaque.[11]

- Children and adolescents who are fed through gastrostomy tubes can still develop calcified deposits on their teeth, which may lead to chronic inflammation in the mouth.[12]

- Children and adolescents with gastric reflux can have enamel erosion similar to that seen with bulimia nervosa.[13]

- Children and adolescents with intellectual and behavioral impairments may be at increased risk for dental caries when they are in behavioral modification programs that use carbohydrate-rich foods as reinforcement.[14]

- Children and adolescents who have difficulty chewing and swallowing may leave more food on their teeth, which can generate plaque.

- Children and adolescents with celiac disease and other gastrointestinal conditions may be at increased risk for tooth malformation and lesions in the mouth.[15]

- Children and adolescents who are fed intra-venously may have premature bone loss.[16]

- Children and adolescents undergoing radiation and chemotherapy are at increased risk for oral disease.[17]

Other Special Considerations

Vitamin Deficiencies

Vitamin A deficiency is believed to contribute to problems in enamel formation and to weaken the epithelial attachment between the teeth and gums, which is a barrier to periodontal infection. Deficiencies of the various forms of vitamin B degrade the oral and surrounding soft tissue with oral ulcers and inflammation of the lip. Vitamin C deficiency causes scurvy and, if untreated, leads to breakdown of the gums and bones. Vitamin D deficiency can affect the enamel quality in developing teeth. Rectifying these deficiencies will reverse damage done to soft tissue and prevent further damage to the teeth.[1]

Fluoride

The widespread availability of fluoride is the primary reason why dental caries among children and adolescents have been significantly reduced in the last several generations. Fluoride increases teeth's resistance to demineralization, encourages the healing of nascent caries, and reduces plaque. The dental professional should determine the appropriate fluoride program on the basis of the child's or adolescent's age, history of and suscepti-

Table 8. Systemic Fluoride Supplements: Recommended Dosage

Age	Fluoride Ion Level in Drinking Water[a]		
	< 0.3 ppm	0.3–0.6 ppm	> 0.6 ppm
Newborn–6 months	None	None	None
6 months–3 years	0.25 mg/day[b]	None	None
3–6 years	0.50 mg/day	0.25 mg/day	None
6–16 years	1.0 mg/day	0.50 mg/day	None

Source: Reprinted from American Dental Association,[18] with permission from ADA Publishing, Inc. Copyright © 1998 American Dental Association.
[a] 1.0 ppm = 1 mg/L.
[b] 2.2 mg sodium fluoride contains 1 mg fluoride ion.

bility to dental caries, and current level of exposure to fluoride.[6(p103–104)]

Children and adolescents receive fluoride in two ways: systemically and topically. Systemic fluorides (i.e., those ingested) include fluoridated water and fluoride supplements (drops, liquids, and tablets). Topical fluorides (i.e., those applied to the surfaces of the teeth) include fluoridated water, fluoride-containing toothpaste, over-the-counter fluoride rinses, and professionally applied fluoride treatments.[6(p103–104)]

Systemic fluorides are very important. Children who drink fluoridated water benefit by incorporating fluoride into their developing teeth. Additionally, people who drink fluoridated water, even adolescents and adults whose teeth are already formed, benefit from the topical effect of fluoride. Today, many families still do not have fluoridated water supplies, and many use multiple sources of water, complicating the delivery of fluoride to children. It is no longer sufficient for the health professional to ask families whether they live in a fluoridated community; it is more appropriate to ask about the source of their drinking and cooking water. If the water is bottled and/or processed, it must be assessed to determine whether the level of fluoride is optimal. Many children and adolescents spend a great deal of time outside the home and drink a mixture of waters, further complicating the delivery of fluoride. Fluoride supplements are recommended only when a child's or adolescent's systemic fluoride ingestion is less than optimal. After the drinking water is assessed and other fluoride sources considered, the health professional can use the information in Table 8 to determine the appropriate supplementation for the child or adolescent.[6(p103–104)]

Topical fluoride is also very important. It is most effective when delivered at very low doses many times a day through water, foods containing fluoride, and fluoridated toothpaste. Almost all toothpaste manufactured in the United States provides topical fluoride.[6(p103–104)]

of age, the addition of foods rich in amino acids (e.g., mashed legumes, lentils, tofu) will provide adequate protein for infants who are consuming a vegan diet.[4]

When energy needs are adequately met through the consumption of a variety of plant foods, protein needs are also likely to be met. When energy supply is inadequate, protein will be used to meet energy needs rather than for tissue synthesis. Because infants and young children have small stomach capacities, small amounts of nutrient-dense foods are recommended five or six times a day. Dairy products and eggs provide high-quality protein. Mixtures of plant proteins also provide balanced, complete sources of amino acids to adequately meet protein requirements.

Metabolic needs can be met by drawing on the body's amino acid pools if a variety of protein-containing foods (as indicated in the Food Guide Pyramid) are eaten throughout the day; consuming precise combinations of plant proteins at the same meal to achieve complete proteins is not necessary.[5] However, foods containing protein in sufficient quality and quantity, or complementary proteins consumed within a few hours of one another, are recommended for infants and children younger than 2 years of age who are not fed breastmilk or infant formula. Soy, amaranth, and quinoa have amino acid patterns similar to those of cow's milk and therefore are important protein sources.

Calcium

Calcium absorption and retention may be 30 to 50 percent higher among vegetarians who consume moderate amounts of protein. Dairy products are excellent sources of calcium. Vegan diets, if not well planned, may contain insufficient calcium. Many vegetarian foods contain moderate amounts of calcium.

Sources of calcium in vegetarian diets include calcium-fortified soy milk, calcium-fortified orange juice, tofu processed with calcium, blackstrap molasses, sesame seeds, tahini (sesame butter), almonds and almond butter, and certain vegetables (e.g., broccoli, okra, collard and mustard greens, kale, rutabaga). Calcium in plant foods that contain high amounts of oxalates (e.g., spinach, Swiss chard, beet greens, rhubarb) is not well absorbed since insoluble calcium oxalate is formed. Fermentation, roasting, and yeasting increase calcium absorption from products (e.g., miso, nuts, leavened bread).[4] Calcium supplements may be necessary if dietary intake is inadequate.

Vitamin D

In addition to calcium, adequate intake of vitamin D is essential for bone health. Although vitamin D can be produced through exposure of the skin to sunlight (20 to 30 minutes two or three times per week), this source of vitamin D cannot be relied on in northern climates during the winter. Dark-skinned persons require longer exposure to sunlight (30 minutes to 3 hours per day) to produce adequate amounts of vitamin D.[4] Sunscreens, smog, and sunlight exposure through glass inhibit vitamin D synthesis.

Breastfed infants who do not have adequate exposure to sunlight should receive a vitamin D supplement (5.0 mg per day); for infants who are not breastfed, soy infant formula provides vitamin D. Children and adolescents can obtain vitamin D from fortified soy milk, fortified breakfast cereals, and fortified margarines.

Vitamin B_{12}

An adequate intake of vitamin B_{12} is essential for growth, red blood cell maturation, and central nervous system functioning. Because of rapid growth and limited nutrient stores in infancy, infants on a vegan diet are at high risk for vitamin B_{12} deficiency, which may be manifested as irritability, apathy, failure to thrive, or developmental regression. Vitamin B_{12} deficiency has been reported in breastfed infants of women on a vegan diet who do not supplement their diet with vitamin B_{12}. If untreated in early stages, vitamin B_{12} deficiency can lead to serious and permanent neurologic damage.[1] High folate intake, which may occur in children and adolescents who follow a vegan diet, can mask hematological changes associated with vitamin B_{12} deficiency, while neurologic damage progresses.

Vitamin B_{12} occurs naturally in animal products, including dairy products and eggs. Although unfortified plant foods (e.g., miso, tempeh, tamari, sauerkraut, seaweed, spirulina, algae) may contain some vitamin B_{12}, it appears to be present in inactive forms, some of which function as antivitamins. Thus, these sources of vitamin B_{12} are considered unreliable.[4]

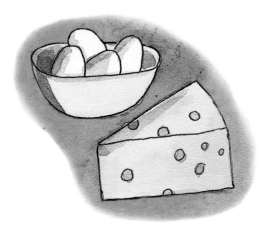

To ensure adequate vitamin B_{12} status, breast-fed infants of women who consume a vegan diet should receive a vitamin B_{12} supplement (0.3 µg per day); if these infants are not breastfed, they should be given soy infant formula. Children and adolescents who consume a vegan diet should receive a vitamin B_{12} supplement or regularly consume one of the following: breakfast cereals, textured soy protein, or soy milk fortified with vitamin B_{12}, or Red Star T-6635+ nutritional yeast flakes.[4]

Iron

Iron needs increase during periods of rapid growth. Although non-heme iron in plant products, dairy foods, and eggs has a lower absorption rate (2 to 20 percent) than that of heme iron in meat, fish, and poultry (15 to 35 percent), vegetarians do not have a higher incidence of iron-deficiency anemia than persons consuming a mixed diet. Iron deficiency has been reported in children fed a macrobiotic diet. The high fiber content of vegetarian diets may make it more difficult for children and adolescents to meet iron needs.

Ascorbic, citric, and malic acid found in fruits and vegetables enhance iron absorption. Foods that decrease iron absorption include wheat bran, nuts, seeds, whole grain cereals, soybeans, spinach, and dairy products. Processes involved in leavening and baking whole grain bread, fermenting soy products (e.g., miso, tempeh), roasting nuts, sprouting seeds, and coagulation with gluconic acid (e.g., tofu) decrease phytates and enhance iron absorption.[4]

Foods high in iron should be consumed daily (e.g., fortified breakfast cereals, instant oatmeal, blackstrap molasses, legumes, tofu, dried fruits, enriched pasta, bread). Iron inhibitors (e.g., coffee, tea, wheat bran) should be avoided.

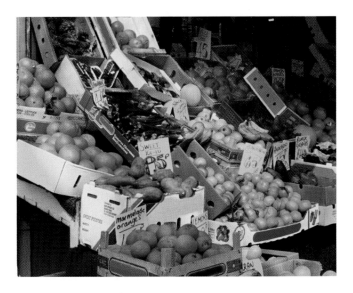

To ensure adequate iron status, breastfed infants should receive a low-dose iron supplement or iron-fortified infant cereal at 6 months of age. Infants on a vegan diet who are not breastfed should receive iron-fortified soy formula for the first 1 to 2 years of life. Children and adolescents should consume juices, fruits, and vegetables high in ascorbic acid daily with meals.

Zinc

Zinc is essential for growth and development. Infants fed breastmilk or soy infant formula will receive adequate amounts of zinc. Milk and eggs are good sources of zinc in lactovegetarian and lacto-ovovegetarian diets. Plant sources of zinc include legumes, tofu, miso, tempeh, nuts, seeds, wheat germ, and whole grains.[4]

To increase the bioavailability of zinc and ensure adequate zinc intake, raw wheat bran should be avoided and the consumption of unleavened bread limited. Legumes should be soaked 1 to 2 hours before cooking, and the water discarded before cooking. Yeast-leavened bread and whole grains, roasted nuts, and sprouted seeds can be used. Because calcium interferes with zinc absorption, consuming calcium supplements with phytate-containing zinc sources (e.g., legumes, nuts, whole grains) should be avoided, but dairy foods are fine in moderation.

Screening and Assessment

The nutritional adequacy of vegetarian and vegan diets can be assessed by asking a few targeted questions. Vegetarian diets vary widely, so it is important to assess precisely what foods are eaten and eliminated from the diet and what supplements are used.

Nutrition Counseling

Vegetarian eating practices need to be carefully planned to provide enough energy, protein, calcium, iron, zinc, and vitamins B_{12} and D. The bioavailability of calcium, iron, and zinc should also be ensured. Careful planning of vegan diets is especially important because it is more difficult to meet nutrient needs from plant foods alone. Parents of infants, children, and adolescents who are vegetarians should be given information on how to plan and provide a nutritionally adequate diet.

When adolescents become vegetarians, parents are often concerned about the diet's nutritional adequacy, especially about meeting protein requirements. Parents need reassurance that a vegetarian diet can meet their adolescent's nutrition needs, and they should receive information on the principles of healthy vegetarian eating for adolescents.

The following guidelines for vegetarian eating practices are based on the references listed at the end of this chapter.

Infancy

- Breastfeed for at least 12 months, and thereafter for as long as the mother and infant wish to continue.

- If breastfeeding is discontinued before 12 months, or breastfeeding occurs fewer than three times a day, feed fortified soy infant formula (20 to 30 oz per day) until the infant is 12 months, or until age 2 if the infant is consuming a vegan diet.

- Avoid cow's milk during the first year of life and low-fat milk during the first 2 years.

- Avoid inappropriate substitutes for breastmilk or infant formula (e.g., unfortified soy milk, rice milk, almond milk, formula prepared from grains).

- Avoid corn syrup or honey.

- Provide a vitamin D supplement to breastfed infants before 6 months of age if their mothers are vitamin D–deficient or if infants are not exposed to adequate sunlight.

- Provide an iron supplement or a supplemental food source of iron (e.g., infant cereal, tofu) for breastfed infants at 4 to 6 months of age.[6]

- Provide a vitamin B_{12} supplement to breastfed infants of mothers who consume a vegan diet.

- Feed nutrient-dense solid foods (e.g., mashed legumes, tofu, cottage or ricotta cheese, yogurt, soy cheese, soy yogurt) at 4 to 6 months of age.

Early Childhood and Middle Childhood

- Provide three meals and two to three snacks per day.

- Avoid bran and excessive intake of bulky foods (e.g., raw fruits and vegetables).

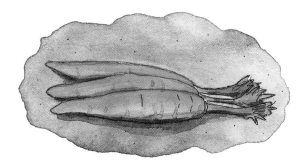

- Encourage eating nutrient-dense foods (e.g., avocado, cheese, soy cheese, hummus, nut butters, tahini, tofu).

- Provide an omega-3 fatty acid source (e.g., canola oil, soy oil, tofu, soybeans, walnuts, wheat germ).

- Avoid excessive restriction of dietary fat.

- Ensure an adequate intake of calcium, zinc, iron, and vitamins B_{12} and D.

Adolescence

- Avoid skipping meals.

- Avoid excessive restriction of dietary fat.

- Limit low-nutrient snacks high in fat and sugar.

- Encourage eating healthy, nutrient-dense snacks (e.g., bagels, bean burritos, falafel, hummus and pita, nachos, nuts, nut butters [almond, cashew,

Table 10. Suggested Daily Food Guide for Lacto-ovovegetarians at Various Intake Levels

Food Groups	Servings per Day, by Age and Daily Caloric Intake			
	1–2 Years (1,300 kcal)	3–6 Years (1,800 kcal)	7–10 Years (2,000 kcal)	11+ Years (2,200–2,800 kcal)
Breads, grains, cereal	5	5	6	9–11
Legumes	1/2	1	1	2–3
Vegetables	2	3	3–5	4–5
Fruits	3	3	4	4
Nuts, seeds	1/2	1/2	1	1
Milk, yogurt, cheese	3	3	3	3
Eggs (limit 3/week)	1/2	1/2	1/2	1/2
Fats, oils (added)	2	4	4	4–6
Sugar (added teaspoons)	3	4	6	6–9

Source: Based in part on Table 3, Haddad.[7]

Note: Serving sizes are based on Haddad.[7]

- Bread, grains, and cereals: 1 slice of bread; 1 biscuit, small roll, pita, tortilla, or muffin; 1/2 bagel, English muffin, or bun; 1/2 cup cooked pasta, rice, quinoa, or couscous; 1/4 cup bulgur; 3/4–1 cup ready-to-eat cereal or 1/2 cup cooked cereal; 4–6 small or 2 large crackers; 1 medium pancake or waffle; 1/3 cup wheat berries; 2 tablespoons wheat germ.
- Legumes: 1/2 cup cooked dry beans (red, navy, kidney, pinto, black, garbanzo, soy); 1/2 cup cooked lentils, split peas, or black-eyed peas; 1/2 cup tofu or tempeh.
- Vegetables: 1/2 cup cooked or 1 cup raw; 3/4 cup juice.
- Fruits: 1 medium piece fresh; 1/2 cup cooked, chopped, or canned; 1/4 cup dried; 3/4 cup juice.
- Nuts and seeds: 1/4 cup; 2 tablespoons nut butter or tahini.
- Milk, yogurt, cheese, or milk alternative: 1 cup milk, yogurt, tofu fortified with calcium, or soy milk fortified with calcium and vitamins B_{12} and D; 1 1/2 oz cheese; 1/2 cup ricotta cheese; 1 1/3 cups cottage cheese.
- Eggs: 1.
- Fats and oils: 1 teaspoon oil, margarine, or mayonnaise; 2 teaspoons salad dressing.
- Sugars: 1 teaspoon sugar, honey, jelly, jam, or syrup.

Table 11. Suggested Daily Food Guide for Vegan Children and Adolescents at Various Intake Levels

Food Groups	Servings per Day, by Age and Daily Caloric Intake			
	1–2 Years (1,300 kcal)	3–6 Years (1,800 kcal)	7–10 Years (2,000 kcal)	11+ Years (2,200–2,800 kcal)
Breads, grains, cereals	5	6	7	10–12
Legumes	1/2	1	1	2–3
Vegetables, dark-green leafy	1	1	1	1
Vegetables, other	1	2	2	3–4
Fruits	2	4	5	4–6
Nuts, seeds	1/2	1/2	1	1
Milk alternatives[a]	3	3	3	3
Fats, oils (added)	2	4	4	4–6
Sugar (added teaspoons)	3	4	6	6–9

Source: Based in part on Table 4, Haddad.[7]

Note: See note to Table 10 for serving sizes.

[a] Fortified with calcium and vitamins B_{12} and D.

peanut, soy], sunflower and pumpkin seeds, tofu dogs, tofu spreads, trail mix, veggie burgers, veggie pizzas, yogurt shakes).

■ Provide an omega-3 fatty acid source (e.g., canola oil, soy oil, tofu, soybeans, walnuts, wheat germ).

■ Ensure an adequate intake of calcium, zinc, iron, and vitamins B_{12} and D.

■ Avoid inappropriate weight-loss practices.

Referral

Referral to a dietitian is helpful in assessing dietary intake and planning healthy vegetarian diets. For infants, children, and adolescents consuming vegetarian diets, referral to a dietitian is essential if the health professional does not have training in or adequate knowledge of nutrition.

References

1. Sanders T. 1995. Vegetarian diets and children. *Pediatric Clinics of North America* 42(4):955–965.

2. U.S. Department of Agriculture and U.S. Department of Health and Human Services. 1995. *Nutrition and Your Health: Dietary Guidelines for Americans* (4th ed.). Washington, DC: U.S. Department of Agriculture.

3. Johnston PK, Haddad EH. 1996. Vegetarian and other dietary practices. In VI Rickert, ed., *Adolescent Nutrition: Assessment and Management.* New York, NY: Chapman and Hall (Aspen Publishers).

4. Melina V, Davis B, Harrison V. 1995. *Becoming Vegetarian: The Complete Guide to Adopting a Healthy Vegetarian Diet.* Summertown, TN: Book Publishing Company.

5. Young V, Pellett P. 1994. Plant proteins in relation to human protein and amino acid nutrition. *American Journal of Clinical Nutrition* 59(Suppl.):1203S–1212S.

6. Centers for Disease Control and Prevention. 1998, April 3. Recommendations to prevent and control iron deficiency in the United States. *Morbidity and Mortality Weekly Report* 47(No. RR-3).

7. Haddad EH. 1994. Development of a vegetarian food guide. *American Journal of Clinical Nutrition* 59(Suppl.):1248S–1254S.

Suggested Reading

Messina M, Messina V. 1996. *The Dietitian's Guide to Vegetarian Diets.* Gaithersburg, MD: Aspen Publishers.

Position of The American Dietetic Association: Vegetarian Diets. 1997. *Journal of The American Dietetic Association* 97(11):1317–1321.

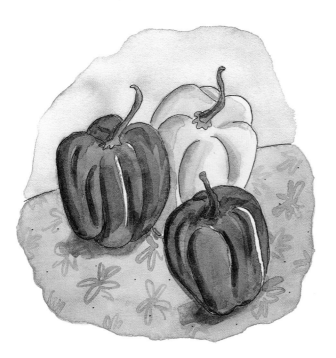

PEDIATRIC UNDERNUTRITION

The terms "pediatric undernutrition" and "failure to thrive" both refer to inadequate growth in young children. When a child's length, weight, or weight-for-length is below the 5th percentile[1] for age and gender on standard growth charts, pediatric undernutrition may be involved. Failure to thrive describes infants and young children who do not grow as expected based on established growth standards for age and gender. Pediatric undernutrition, sometimes used as a synonym for failure to thrive, refers specifically to growth impairment. Often assumed to be a disorder of medical origin (organic failure to thrive) or psychosocial origin (nonorganic failure to thrive), pediatric undernutrition is likely to originate from a combination of medical, psychosocial, economic, and policy factors.

Undernutrition typically occurs in the first 3 years of life and can often be identified around age 1 by careful monitoring of the infant's growth. Assessment and treatment should begin as soon as the problem is identified.

Approximately 3 to 5 percent of young children in the United States meet the growth criteria for undernutrition,[1] although the prevalence may be higher in some communities; some of these children are growing normally, but all warrant assessment.

Significance

Pediatric undernutrition may impair a child's optimal growth and development into adulthood. The condition is also associated with diminished immunologic resistance, decreased physical activity, and long-term problems in cognitive development, academic performance, and socio-affective competence. These effects are of greater concern if the undernutrition is severe or occurs during infancy, when brain growth is most rapid. However, undernourished infants and children can benefit from intervention that includes improved nutrition.

Contextual Issues

Health professionals need to work closely with families when pediatric undernutrition is a concern, because issues can be complex and require extra time. A health professional should observe the infant or young child eating. Ideally, the meal can be videotaped and the tape reviewed with the parents in a supportive way to provide anticipatory guidance about feeding. Home visits by dietitians, nurses, or other health professionals can increase their understanding of the family's lifestyle and enhance their ability to advise the family.

Biological and Developmental

Infants born with low birthweight are likely to continue to be small and to require extra care with nutrition to ensure that they have the best possible opportunity to grow and develop. Special growth charts are available to monitor their growth.

In addition to low birthweight, a diagnosis of inadequate growth may derive from familial patterns of normal growth (e.g., parents who are short or thin, or who experienced delayed growth and sexual maturation). Inadequate growth may also result from medical conditions (e.g., otitis media, diarrhea) and a wide variety of uncommon conditions, most of which can be identified after a careful medical history and physical examination. Zinc deficiency (common in undernourished children) should be treated, and children should be screened for iron-deficiency anemia and treated if it is present.

A few children may have trouble swallowing (manifested by gagging, excessive drooling, and other symptoms) and may require help from an occupational therapist or speech-language pathologist. In addition to undernutrition, some children have delays in speech and language or other aspects of development and should be referred to early intervention programs.

Behavioral and Familial

Food choice may be another factor that contributes to impaired nutrition in children. Some cases of undernutrition have been associated with excessive intake of fruit juice. In children with chronic diarrhea, it is helpful to obtain a dietary history, including the volume of fruit juice consumed. Parents can begin to assess this factor by keeping a 3-day food diary and asking a dietitian or other health professional to review it to determine whether the child's food intake is well balanced and contains sufficient calories, protein, and fat necessary to sustain growth. (Fat should not be restricted in the first 2 years of life.) Health professionals can learn about the frequency and regularity of the feedings by reviewing the family's food diary and asking the parents to describe a typical day. (For further information about eating behaviors, see the Infancy and Early Childhood chapters.)

Cultural, Economic, and Psychosocial

Cultural beliefs affect many aspects of infant and early childhood nutrition (e.g., breastfeeding and weaning, expectations about the child's weight, family food preferences, ways to deal with the child's independence). Health professionals need to listen attentively, become aware of their own assumptions, and be open to the practices of other cultures. They may also observe cultural differences in professional-parent relationships, learn to negotiate culturally based disagreements, and learn new languages or use interpreters. (For further information about culture and food choices, see the Cultural Awareness for Nutrition Counseling chapter.)

Health professionals should try to sensitively determine whether the family has enough money and other resources (e.g., transportation) to obtain food. Federal food assistance and nutrition programs can provide a substantial part of an infant's or child's daily nutrition requirements. (See Appendix K: Federal Food Assistance and Nutrition Programs.) Food shelves and pantries, churches and other places of worship, and businesses can also provide food.

Much of what health professionals do is factual: They obtain information and provide anticipatory guidance. For many families, this educational approach is sufficient; for others, a psychosocial approach may be needed. If health professionals feel frustrated and worried about a family, their feelings may be a sign that more than guidance is needed. Family stressors, psychological issues, or a disturbance in the parent-child relationship may need to be addressed. In these instances, both the health professional and the family can benefit from the services of a mental health professional. If the parents fail to follow through with the recommended guidance and the health professional suspects neglect, it may be necessary to contact protective services.

Treatment and Management

Because multiple factors can be involved in helping an infant or child with undernutrition, several professionals—dietitians, nurses, other health professionals, child care providers, and specialists in child development or mental health—may be needed. They must learn to understand and embrace both the individuality and the complexity that children and families present. Ideally, these professionals work as a team; however, in many communities they work in different agencies. Coordination among agencies in the community is a significant challenge that must be addressed. It is important

that they work closely with one another and with families to share understanding and information and to plan effective interventions. They can also work at the interagency level to coordinate services and to identify gaps and deficiencies that require additional help.

Reference

1. Kessler DB, Dawson P, eds. 1999. *Failure to Thrive and Pediatric Undernutrition: A Transdisciplinary Approach.* Baltimore, MD: Paul H. Brookes Publishing Company.

Suggested Reading

Peterson KE. 1993. Failure to thrive. In PM Queen, CE Lang, eds., *Handbook of Pediatric Nutrition.* Gaithersburg, MD: Aspen Publishers.

Satter E. 1987. *How to Get Your Kid to Eat—But Not Too Much: From Birth to Adolescence.* Palo Alto, CA: Bull Publishing Company.

IRON-DEFICIENCY ANEMIA

Iron-deficiency anemia typically involves red blood cells that are abnormally small in size, with decreased hemoglobin or hematocrit, and a reduced capacity to deliver oxygen to body cells and tissues. In 1998, the Centers for Disease Control and Prevention (CDC) updated the criteria for defining anemia in a healthy reference population (Table 12). The distribution of hemoglobin and hematocrit values for iron-deficiency anemia differs in children and adolecents and in males and females.

High altitudes and cigarette smoking increase iron-deficiency anemia cutpoints (see Table 13).

Table 12. Maximum Hemoglobin Concentration and Hematocrit Values for Iron-Deficiency Anemia[a]

Sex/Age, Years	Hemoglobin, < g/dL	Hematocrit, < %
Males and Females		
1 to < 2[b]	11.0	32.9
2 to < 5	11.1	33.0
5 to < 8	11.5	34.5
8 to < 12	11.9	35.4
Males		
12 to < 15	12.5	37.3
15 to < 18	13.3	39.7
≥ 18	13.5	39.9
Females[c]		
12 to < 15	11.8	35.7
15 to <18	12.0	35.9
≥ 18	12.0	35.7

Source: Adapted from Table 6, Centers for Disease Control and Prevention.[1]

[a] Age- and sex-specific cutoff values for anemia are based on the 5th percentile from the third National Health and Nutrition Examination Survey (NHANES III).

[b] Although no data are available from NHANES III to determine the maximum hemoglobin concentration and hematocrit values for anemia among infants, the values listed for children ages 1 to < 2 years can be used for infants ages 6 to 12 months.

[c] Nonpregnant and lactating adolescents.

Table 13. Adjustment of Maximum Hemoglobin Concentration and Hematocrit Values for Iron-Deficiency Anemia

	Hemoglobin Concentration, < g/dL	Hematocrit, %
Altitude, feet		
3,000–3,999	+0.2	+0.5
4,000–4,999	+0.3	+1.0
5,000–5,999	+0.5	+1.5
6,000–6,999	+0.7	+2.0
7,000–7,999	+1.0	+3.0
8,000–8,999	+1.3	+4.0
9,000–9,999	+1.6	+5.0
10,000–11,000	+2.0	+6.0
Cigarette smoking		
0.5 to < 1.0 pack per day	+0.3	+1.0
1.0 to < 2.0 packs per day	+0.5	+1.5
≥ 2.0 packs per day	+0.7	+2.0
All smokers	+0.3[a]	+1.0

Source: Reproduced from Table 7, Centers for Disease Control and Prevention.[1]

[a] In place of the adjustments based on packs per day, a single hemoglobin concentration adjustment of 0.3 g/dL may be used for all smokers.

Altitudes above 3,000 feet raise the cutpoint for iron-deficiency anemia because of lower oxygen partial pressure, a reduction in oxygen saturation of blood, and an increase in red cell production. Cigarette smoking also raises the cutpoint for iron-deficiency anemia because carboxyhemoglobin formed from carbon monoxide during smoking has no oxygen-carrying capacity.

Significance

Iron deficiency is the most prevalent form of nutrition deficiency in this country. The risk of iron-deficiency anemia is highest during infancy and adolescence because of the increased iron requirements from rapid growth. In healthy full-term infants, iron stores are adequate until age 4 to 6 months. Iron requirements may exceed dietary iron intake after this time. The onset of menarche and low dietary iron intake also contribute to a higher risk of iron-deficiency anemia among adolescent females. Iron-deficiency anemia is more common in populations with low incomes.

Iron-deficiency anemia has been associated with delayed psychomotor development, cognitive deficits, and behavioral disturbances in young children. Iron-deficiency anemia has also been associated with impaired growth and development, depression of the immune system, fatigue, decreased resistance to infection, decreased physical performance, decreased levels of endurance, reduced attention span, decreased school performance, and increased susceptibility to lead poisoning. Among pregnant adolescents and women, iron deficiency in early gestation may increase the risk of giving birth to a preterm or low-birthweight infant.[1]

Risk Factors

Increased demand for iron, decreased intake of iron, and/or greater loss of iron from the body are associated with a higher risk of iron-deficiency anemia. The following conditions are associated with an increased risk of developing iron-deficiency anemia:

- Periods of rapid growth
- Preterm or low-birthweight birth
- Low dietary intake of meat, fish, poultry, or foods rich in ascorbic acid
- Macrobiotic diets
- Inappropriate consumption of cow's milk (infants should not consume cow's milk; children should not consume more than 24 oz of cow's milk per day)

- Use of non–iron-fortified infant formula for more than 2 months
- Exclusive breastfeeding after age 6 months without the addition of iron-fortified supplemental foods in the infant's diet
- Meal skipping, frequent dieting
- Pregnancy
- Participation in endurance sports (e.g., long-distance running, swimming, cycling)
- Intensive physical training
- Recent blood loss, recent pregnancy, heavy/lengthy menstrual periods
- Chronic use of aspirin or nonsteroidal anti-inflammatory drugs (e.g., ibuprofen)
- Parasitic infections

Screening

Following are the CDC recommendations for iron-deficiency anemia screening (based on the hemoglobin and hematocrit values in Table 12).[1]

Infants and Children Ages 1 to 5

Health professionals should assess all infants and children for risk of iron-deficiency anemia.[1] Those at high risk or those with known risk factors need to be screened for iron-deficiency anemia with a standard laboratory test.

Universal Screening (Those at High Risk)

At 9 to 12 months, 6 months later (at 15 to 18 months), and annually from ages 2 to 5 years, screen those at high risk for iron-deficiency anemia, including

- Infants and children in families with low incomes

- Infants and children who are eligible for WIC

- Infants and children who are migrants or recently arrived refugees

Selective Screening (Those with Known Risk Factors)

In populations of infants and children not at high risk, screen only those individuals who have known risk factors for iron-deficiency anemia.

Before age 6 months, screen preterm and low-birthweight infants who are fed infant formula that is not fortified with iron.

At 9 to 12 months, and 6 months later (at 15 to 18 months), screen the following:

- Infants born preterm or with low birthweight

- Infants fed non–iron-fortified infant formula for more than 2 months

- Infants fed cow's milk before 12 months of age

- Breastfed infants who do not receive adequate iron from supplemental foods after 6 months of age

- Children who consume more than 24 oz of cow's milk per day

- Children with special health care needs who use medications that interfere with iron absorption (e.g., antacids, calcium, phosphorus, magnesium), or those with chronic infection, inflam-matory disorders, restricted diets, or extensive blood loss from a wound, an accident, or surgery

At ages 2 to 5 years, annually screen the following:

- Children who consume a diet low in iron

- Children with limited access to food because of poverty or neglect

- Children with special health care needs

Children Ages 5 to 12 and Adolescent Males Ages 12 to 18

Screen only those with known risk factors (e.g., low iron intake, special health care needs, previous diagnosis of iron-deficiency anemia).

Adolescent Males Ages 18 to 21

Adolescents 18 or older should be screened if risk factors are present.

Adolescent Females Ages 12 to 21

Screen annually those with known risk factors (e.g., extensive menstrual or other blood loss, low iron intake, a previous diagnosis of iron-deficiency anemia).

Screen every 5 to 10 years during routine health examinations.

Diagnosis and Treatment

Low hemoglobin values should be confirmed by a repeat hemoglobin or hematocrit test. This is especially true when screening with capillary samples (fingerstick), because of the reported variability in capillary samples.

Parents of infants, children, and adolescents should receive information on the treatment of iron-deficiency anemia. Treating iron deficiency involves both iron therapy and improving eating behaviors. After anemia of dietary origin has been treated successfully, recurrence can be prevented with an improved diet.

Iron Therapy

If low hemoglobin is confirmed, the following treatment is recommended:[1]

- Infants and children younger than 5 years: 3 mg/kg body weight of elemental iron drops per day

- Children ages 5 to 12 years: one 60-mg elemental iron tablet per day

- Adolescent males ages 12 to 18 years: two 60-mg elemental iron tablets per day

- Adolescent females ages 12 to 18 years: one to two 60-mg elemental iron tablets per day

Iron preparations are absorbed most effectively when taken between meals or at bedtime. If gastrointestinal intolerance (e.g., nausea, cramping, diarrhea, constipation) occurs, iron can be taken with meals. Tolerance may also be improved by using a lower dosage, gradually increasing the dosage, or using a different form (e.g., ferrous gluconate). Since iron absorption occurs primarily in the duodenum, timed-release iron preparations may be less effectively absorbed. Iron preparations should not be taken within 1 hour of substances that may inhibit iron absorption (e.g., dairy products, casein, antacids, calcium supplements, coffee, tea, bran, whole grains). To prevent accidental poisoning, iron preparations should be stored out of the reach of infants and children.

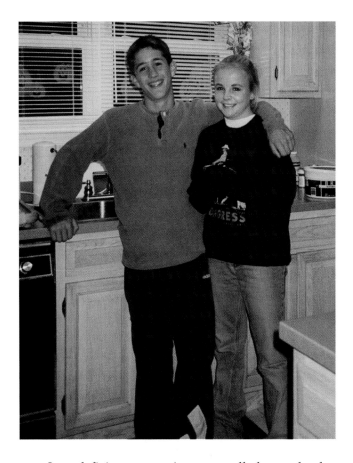

Iron-deficiency anemia can usually be resolved effectively through 6 to 8 weeks of treatment with ferrous sulfate. If the hemoglobin does not respond to iron therapy (increase of 1 g within approximately 1 month), iron deficiency should be confirmed by a serum ferritin determination. Values less than or equal to 15 µg/L in infants older than 6 months, children, and adolescents indicate depleted iron stores. Ferritin values may be falsely elevated when infection or inflammation is present. Serum transferrin-receptor concentration may be a more reliable indicator of iron stores because it is not influenced by chronic infection, inflammation, or disease.[1,2] To replace iron stores, iron therapy should be continued for an additional 3 months after the hemoglobin has returned to normal (i.e., when serum ferritin is greater than 15 µg/L).

Dietary Strategies

Dietary strategies can improve iron status and help prevent recurrence of iron-deficiency anemia.

Iron status can be improved through increased consumption of lean meat, fish, and poultry, which contain heme, an effectively absorbed form of iron from hemoglobin and myoglobin; meat, fish, and poultry also enhance absorption of the less-bioavailable plant sources of iron (e.g., grains, dried peas and beans, spinach).

Sources of vitamin C (e.g., citrus and fortified fruit juices, citrus fruit, strawberries, cantaloupe, green peppers, broccoli, cabbage) taken with meals increase the absorption of nonmeat sources of iron by maintaining the iron in its reduced, more soluble form. The use of highly fortified breakfast cereals can also improve iron intake. Liver is not recommended because of its high cholesterol content and potentially high level of environmental toxins.

Nutrition Counseling

Primary prevention of iron deficiency should be achieved through diet. The following general guidelines are based on CDC recommendations for preventing iron-deficiency anemia in infants, children, and adolescents.[1]

Infancy

- Breastfeed throughout the first year of life, with exclusive breastfeeding for the first 4 to 6 months (without supplementary liquid, formula, or food).

- When exclusive breastfeeding is stopped, provide a supplemental source of iron (approximately 1 mg/kg body weight per day), preferably from supplementary foods.

- Use iron-fortified infant formula for infants who are not breastfed or who are partially breastfed.

- Provide iron supplement (2 to 4 mg of iron drops per kg body weight per day, not to exceed 15 mg per day) for preterm or low-birthweight breastfed infants, beginning at age 1 month and continuing through age 12 months.

- Encourage use of only breastmilk or iron-fortified infant formula for any milk-based part of the diet and discourage use of low-iron milk (e.g., cow's, goat's, soy) for infants.

- Provide iron-containing foods when exclusive breastfeeding is stopped (e.g., 4 tablespoons [dry measure, before adding milk[3]] of iron-fortified infant cereal per day).

- Supplement with iron drops (1 mg per kg body weight per day) for breastfed infants who receive insufficient iron from foods by age 6 months.

- Encourage one feeding per day of foods rich in vitamin C by age 6 months.

- Introduce plain, pureed meats after age 6 months or when the infant is developmentally ready to consume such foods.

Early Childhood, Middle Childhood, and Adolescence

▪ Children ages 1 to 5 years should consume no more than 24 oz of cow's, goat's, or soy milk per day.

▪ Include sources of iron-rich foods (e.g., fortified breakfast cereals, meat, fish, poultry) and vitamin C–rich foods (e.g., citrus and fortified fruit juices, citrus fruit, strawberries, cantaloupe, green peppers, broccoli, cabbage) to enhance iron absorption.

▪ Limit snacks that are low in nutrients.

▪ Avoid skipping meals or chronic dieting.

▪ Limit coffee, tea, and colas.

Referral

Referral to a dietitian is helpful in cases of severe or prolonged iron-deficiency anemia. All infants, children, and pregnant or lactating adolescents who are eligible should be referred to WIC. (See Appendix J: Nutrition Resources.)

References

1. Centers for Disease Control and Prevention. 1998, April 3. Recommendations to prevent and control iron deficiency in the United States. *MMWR* 47 (No. RR-3).

2. Cook JD. 1994. Iron-deficiency anaemia. *Bailliere's Clinical Haematology* 7(4):787–804.

3. Fomon SJ, ed. 1993. *Nutrition of Normal Infants*. St. Louis, MO: Mosby-Year Book.

FOOD ALLERGY

The term "food allergy" is often misused. Only about 5 percent of all adverse reactions to foods and food additives in the general population are true allergies.[1] Generally, there are two broad categories of adverse reactions to foods: food allergy/hypersensitivity, and food intolerance.[2]

Food allergy/hypersensitivity refers to a condition in which a person's immune system responds to the ingestion of a particular food protein. (This reaction may or may not be mediated by immunoglobulin E [IgE].) Trace amounts of the allergenic food may be sufficient to trigger an adverse reaction. Symptoms can occur within seconds or as long as 72 hours after exposure and can include itching, hives, rash (eczema), vomiting, diarrhea, abdominal pain, or swelling of the lips, tongue, and face.

All non–immune-mediated reactions to foods are referred to as food intolerance. This condition includes (a) intolerance because of a lack of an essential enzyme (e.g., lactose intolerance); (b) reactions to pharmacologically active chemicals in foods (e.g., MSG); (c) reactions to naturally occurring pharmacologically active agents in foods (e.g., phenylethylamine in chocolate); and (d) reactions to toxic compounds in foods (e.g., aflatoxin). The adverse response is usually dose-dependent.

The terms "food sensitivity" and "adverse reaction to food" are synonymous and may be used to describe either immune-mediated or non–immune-mediated responses to food.

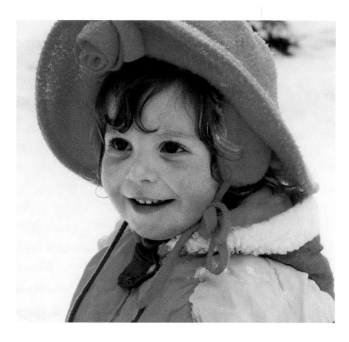

Significance

Food allergies are particularly prevalent in infants and children because their digestive and immune systems are still immature.[1,3] As children mature, food allergies are often outgrown. Food allergies diagnosed in children are more likely to be outgrown than those diagnosed in older children. However, the more severe the initial reaction to the food, the longer it takes for the child to become tolerant of the food.[2] Some food allergies are lifelong.

Three nutrition-related issues emerge with food allergies. First, food allergies may be greatly reduced or delayed in children when families at high risk for food allergies are identified through screening and when appropriate dietary and environmental measures are taken early in the child's life.[4,5] Second, the most effective means of preventing adverse reactions and developing tolerance is removing the

they will be less likely to perceive the avoidance as a restriction imposed by their parents. The health professional can discuss the food allergy with the older child or adolescent and do controlled challenges, if medically appropriate, so that he or she recognizes the adverse effects and understands the need to avoid the food.

Referral

Families of children and adolescents with food allergies can be referred to organizations such as the Food Allergy Network. (See Appendix J: Nutrition Resources.)

References

1. Perkin JE. 1990. *Food Allergies and Adverse Reactions.* Gaithersburg, MD: Aspen Publishers.

2. Anderson JA. 1994. Tips when considering the diagnosis of food allergy. *Topics in Clinical Nutrition* 9(3):11–21.

3. Joneja JV. 1995. *Managing Food Allergy and Intolerances: A Practical Guide.* West Vancouver, British Columbia, Canada: McQuaid Consulting Group.

4. Metcalfe DD, Sampson HA, Simon RA. 1991. *Food Allergy: Adverse Reactions to Foods and Food Additives.* Boston, MA: Blackwell Scientific Publications.

5. Kendall PA, Gloeckner JW. 1994. Managing food allergies and sensitivities. *Topics in Clinical Nutrition* 9(3):1–10.

6. Satter E. 1995. Feeding dynamics: Helping children to eat well. *Journal of Pediatric Health Care* 9(4):178–184.

7. Carroll P. 1994. Guidelines for counseling patients with food sensitivities. *Topics in Clinical Nutrition* 9(3):33–37.

Suggested Reading

Sampson HA, Burks AW. 1996. Mechanism of food allergy. *Annual Review of Nutrition* 16:161–177.

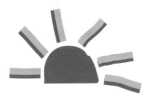

Managing a Child's Severe Food Allergy

Miya Kim is 4 years old and about to start a half-day preschool program that meets three times a week. Miya's mother is apprehensive because Miya has serious allergic reactions to some foods. When Miya was 6 months old, she ate a spoonful of mashed potatoes that contained milk and cheddar cheese; she immediately developed hives and within minutes had difficulty breathing. Miya was rushed to the hospital, where she was diagnosed with a severe allergy to cow's milk. So far, it has been determined that she is allergic to milk and other dairy products, peanuts, and shellfish. Mrs. Kim has learned how to treat Miya's anaphylactic reactions (severe allergic reactions) with a shot of epinephrine and an antihistamine.

Because of the severity of Miya's allergic reactions, her mother has monitored Miya's food intake very carefully. Mrs. Kim is concerned that when Miya begins the preschool program, she will be exposed to allergenic foods that may be served as a classroom snack.

Mrs. Kim discusses her concerns with a dietitian, Sue Panzarine, at her preschool screening visit. Ms. Panzarine tells Mrs. Kim that she can understand her concerns. She is pleased to learn that Mrs. Kim has taught Miya how to ask about ingredients in the foods she is offered, and that Mrs. Kim and her daughter have practiced these skills at restaurants and friends' homes. Miya also understands the symptoms of her allergic reactions and knows the importance of telling an adult as soon as the symptoms occur. Ms. Panzarine shows Mrs. Kim a videotape for parents that explains food allergies and how to treat them. She suggests that Mrs. Kim meet with the teachers and program director at the preschool to discuss these concerns and to show the videotape to Miya's teachers.

One week before preschool is scheduled to begin, Mrs. Kim meets with the teachers and program director to discuss Miya's needs. Together, they view the videotape on allergic reactions and Mrs. Kim explains how to treat an anaphylactic reaction.

Mrs. Kim also gives the staff a list of snack foods that are safe for Miya and a list of allergenic ingredients of concern.

On the first day of class, Miya and her mother arrive early. Mrs. Kim meets with the other parents and gives each of them a letter that introduces Miya and explains her food allergies. Mrs. Kim stays during the first class to answer questions from the teachers and parents. She is reassured to discover that everyone is willing to ensure a safe and healthy learning environment for Miya.

DIABETES MELLITUS

Diabetes mellitus is a chronic disease in which the body does not produce or properly use insulin. Insulin is a hormone manufactured by the beta cells of the pancreas that the body requires to maximally use glucose from digested food as an energy source. Diabetes mellitus is characterized by elevated glucose in the blood and urine. The goal of treatment is to manage the factors that affect blood glucose levels (e.g., insulin, food, and physical activity) to promote near-normal levels. Although the exact cause of diabetes is not known, a genetic component to the disease is recognized; environmental and immunologic factors may also play roles.

There are two main types of diabetes mellitus. In type 1 diabetes mellitus, the body does not produce any insulin, and daily insulin injections are required. Type 1 occurs in infants, children, adolescents, and young adults and accounts for 5 to 10 percent of all cases of diabetes mellitus.[1] In contrast, persons with type 2 diabetes mellitus continue to produce insulin, but the body is unable to make enough or properly use what is made.

Type 2 has typically been diagnosed after the age of 40 and accounts for 90 to 95 percent of all cases of diabetes mellitus; however, because of the increasing prevalence of childhood obesity, the number of children and adolescents with type 2 is increasing. Treatment of type 2 includes lifestyle changes to promote weight management and regular physical activity, as well as oral medications or supplemental insulin if needed. Prevention of type 2 diabetes mellitus involves the promotion of a healthy weight and a regular physical activity program to improve carbohydrate metabolism and insulin sensitivity. (See the Obesity chapter.) This chapter will focus on type 1 diabetes mellitus.

Significance

Over 700,000 people in the United States have type 1 diabetes mellitus; it affects about 1 in every 600 children.[2] The quality of care that children and adolescents receive may affect their long-term health. Control of diabetes mellitus aims to prevent acute complications (e.g., diabetic ketoacidosis and severe hypoglycemia, which may be life threatening) and chronic microvascular and macrovascular complications, which can lead to blindness, kidney disease, nerve damage, amputations, heart disease, and stroke.

Nutritional Adequacy

The treatment of type 1 diabetes mellitus involves careful attention to insulin administration, food intake, and physical activity to promote acceptable blood glucose and lipid levels. Most children and adolescents receive a mixed dose of short- and intermediate-acting insulin twice a day, before breakfast and before the evening meal. Multiple insulin regimens that use short-acting insulin before each meal and a longer-acting insulin once or twice a day may also be used to help improve diabetes mellitus control. Blood glucose monitoring two to four times a day is recommended to help identify blood glucose patterns and to adjust insulin or food intake.

The goals of medical management and nutrition therapy include continued normal growth and development, sexual maturation, reduction of hyperglycemic and hypoglycemic episodes, promotion of healthy eating and physical activity, and improvement of overall health and diabetes mellitus control to reduce the risk or delay the progression of complications.

Specific guidelines for energy intake vary with the age of the child or adolescent and should be individualized on the basis of an in-depth nutritional assessment and nutrition and physical activity history. Energy requirements should initially be based on the child's or adolescent's typical food intake, pattern of growth, level of physical activity, and estimated energy allowance for age and sex.[3] A child or adolescent who has lost weight before diagnosis often requires additional energy for catch-up weight gain. The distribution of calories should be individualized according to desired glucose, lipid, and weight goals, but it should still be similar to those recommended for the entire population to promote a healthier lifestyle (approximately 55 to 60 percent carbohydrates, 10 to 20 percent protein, and 30 percent or less fat).[4]

Sucrose substituted for other carbohydrates does not promote adverse hyperglycemia in persons with diabetes mellitus; therefore, foods containing sucrose are allowed in moderation, and the variety of foods permitted in diabetic meal plans has increased.[4] Nutrition inadequacies may result from food intolerance or personal food preferences (e.g., lactose intolerance, vegetarian eating practices). For these circumstances, the dietitian needs to provide nutrition counseling about healthy food choices and appropriate alternatives.

Screening

No screening recommendations for the diagnosis of diabetes mellitus in children or adolescents have been established. During the early course of type 1 diabetes mellitus, children and adolescents may present with symptoms of polyuria, polydipsia, polyphagia, and weight loss. At this time, a random blood glucose level over 200 mg/dL (11.1 mmol/L) or a fasting plasma glucose over 126 mg/dL (7.0 mmol/L) is sufficient to make the diagnosis.[5] Early diagnosis reduces the risk of more dangerous conditions (e.g., increased weight loss, dehydration, diabetic ketoacidosis).

Nutrition Counseling

Nutrition counseling is essential to the effective self-management of diabetes mellitus and should be presented in stages.[2] Younger children will depend on a family member to administer insulin and monitor blood glucose levels, food intake, and physical activity. The daily tasks of diabetes mellitus management should be taught gradually, and the responsibility for care should be shared with the maturing older child or adolescent.

Initial nutrition counseling is provided at diagnosis and prepares the child or adolescent and family for living with diabetes mellitus. During this stage, the family should be taught basic management skills (e.g., insulin administration, blood glucose monitoring, meal and snack planning). Nutrition counseling should focus on eating meals and snacks at consistent times every day, being consistent in the amount of carbohydrates eaten at each meal and snack, learning to identify food groups and portion sizes, and knowing how to recognize and treat low blood-glucose levels. Explain-

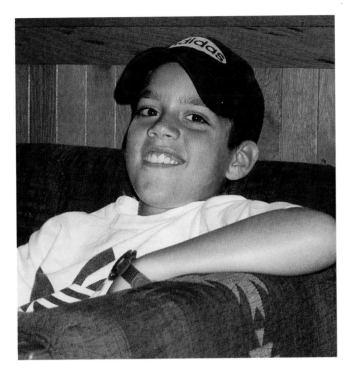

ing the use of a snack system that provides a variety of foods is an effective teaching tool at this time and demonstrates to the family how favorite foods can be incorporated into the meal plan.[6] Other recommended educational materials for the initial and subsequent stages are available from the American Diabetes Association and The American Dietetic Association.[7–10]

Once the child (if old enough) or adolescent and family demonstrate a basic understanding of diabetes mellitus and can follow the day-to-day tasks required for its control, nutrition counseling should be offered to teach insulin adjustment, expand food choices, and allow flexibility in scheduling meals and physical activity. The family can be given guidelines on adjusting the dose of short-acting insulin when necessary and on varying food intake and physical activity. The dietitian can provide nutrition counseling on eating away from home, buying school lunches, eating at fast-food and other restaurants, converting nutrient information on food labels to exchanges or carbohydrate equivalents, increasing food intake for increased physical activity, and planning sick-day meals.

Counseling for intensive diabetes mellitus management should be provided to those who demonstrate competency in daily management and are highly motivated to achieve near-normal blood glucose levels.[11] The focus at this stage is blood-glucose pattern identification and evaluation and the promotion of increasingly sophisticated decision-making about adjusting insulin, food intake, and physical activity. The dietitian can provide more information about the effect of food on blood glucose levels, ways to estimate carbohydrate intake more precisely, and ways to calculate carbohydrate-to-insulin ratios. Because the documented side effects of improved glucose control are an increase in hypoglycemic episodes and unwanted weight gain, intensive nutrition counseling should also include guidance on preventing and managing low blood sugar and managing weight.

Infancy

Infants are dependent on parents to manage their diabetes. Because they cannot communicate when they experience symptoms of hypoglycemia, blood glucose goals are more liberal (100 to 220 mg/dL). Hypoglycemia should be first treated by giving the infant one-half of a carbohydrate serving (e.g., 2 oz apple juice), but more may be given if the infant's blood glucose is still low after 15 minutes. Breastmilk or infant formula is recommended throughout the first year of life, and new supplemental foods and textures should be introduced as appropriate. Parents should be taught how to read nutrition labels to determine the carbohydrate content of infant formula and baby foods (e.g., one carbohydrate serving equals 15 g carbohydrate). Rapid-acting insulin is often given after feeding to offset the infant's food intake.

Early Childhood

Children are at a stage when they may exert their independence by refusing to eat certain foods or meals, and the amount and variety of food eaten may vary considerably depending on food habits, changes in routines, and level of physical activity. Younger children may also have difficulty recognizing and verbally labeling symptoms of hypoglycemia; therefore, blood glucose goals are usually higher for this age group than for older children.

With a focus on the child's consistency of carbohydrate intake, the dietitian can provide meal patterns that specify the number of carbohydrate servings and ranges for meat and fat exchanges. Families should be taught that, in terms of the carbohydrate content of food exchanges, one bread exchange equals one fruit exchange equals one milk exchange. This information helps increase food choices and may avert food battles and rejection of food. The families should also be advised that most toddlers have at least three snacks per day, and flexibility in food choices will help ensure the toddler's cooperation.

Middle Childhood

Children become more emotionally independent between the ages of 7 and 12 years. Motor, reading, math, and reasoning skills increase quickly, as do independence and pride in one's accomplishments. Eating at school needs to be managed carefully to promote the child's sense of well-being:

Children want to eat what the other children are eating. The dietitian can help plan a meal pattern for lunch that matches the standard lunch served at school. The dietitian can also recommend convenient, favorite foods for snacks at school (e.g., granola bars, crackers, cookies) to promote consistency of food intake. On gym days, an extra snack should be provided before the physical activity to help prevent exercise-induced hypoglycemia. However, this additional carbohydrate may not be necessary if the child's blood glucose level is greater than 100 mg/dL.[12] It is often helpful for the dietitian to collaborate with school personnel (e.g., teachers, food service workers) to explain the dietary management goals for the child.

Adolescence

Adolescence is a time for further developing one's sense of identity and increasing autonomy and independence. More time is spent with friends, and the family's influence is diminished. Because social activities often revolve around food, adolescents with type 1 diabetes mellitus need a flexible meal plan that permits choice and spontaneity. Snacks may be omitted in the morning and the afternoon depending on blood glucose levels, physical activity, and weight management goals. However, the evening snack should always be kept to help decrease the risk of hypoglycemia during the night. The risk of eating disorders needs to be recognized and addressed; adolescents with diabetes mellitus may try to manage their weight by reducing or skipping their insulin. Older adolescents with varying work and school schedules may decide to begin the more flexible multiple daily insulin-injection regimens. This intensification of management will need to be coordinated with the health professional, and additional education about carbohydrates and insulin adjustment will need to be provided.

Referral

Referral to an interdisciplinary, pediatric diabetes-mellitus management program with a pediatric endocrinologist, nurse, dietitian, and social worker should be considered at diagnosis for these groups: infants and young children; older children and adolescents with frequent hospitalizations for ketoacidosis or severe hypoglycemia; children, adolescents, and/or families with psychosocial problems; and those who are using multiple daily insulin injections for improved glucose control.

References

1. American Diabetes Association. 1994. *Maximizing the Role of Nutrition in Diabetes Management: Highlights of a Clinical Education Program.* Alexandria, VA: American Diabetes Association.

2. Connell JE, Thomas-Dobersen D. 1991. Nutritional management of children and adolescents with insulin-dependent diabetes mellitus: A review by the Diabetes Care and Education Dietetic Practice Group. *Journal of The American Dietetic Association* 91(12):1556–1564.

3. National Research Council, Commission on Life Sciences, Food and Nutrition Board, Subcommittee on the Tenth Edition of the RDAs. 1989. *Recommended Dietary Allowances* (10th ed.). Washington, DC: National Academy Press.

4. Nutrition recommendations and principles for people with diabetes mellitus. 1994. *Journal of The American Dietetic Association* 94(5):504–506.

5. Report of the Expert Committee on the Diagnosis and Classification of Diabetes Mellitus. 1997. *Diabetes Care* 20(7):1183–1197.

6. Loghmani E, Rickard KA. 1994. Alternative snack system for children and teenagers with diabetes mellitus. *Journal of The American Dietetic Association* 94(10):1145–1148.

7. American Diabetes Association, The American Dietetic Association. 1995. *Exchange Lists for Meal Planning.* Alexandria, VA: American Diabetes Association; Chicago, IL: The American Dietetic Association.

8. Daly A, Barry B, Gillespie S, Kulkarnie K, Richardson M. 1995. *Carbohydrate Counting: Getting Started.* Alexandria, VA: American Diabetes Association; Chicago, IL: The American Dietetic Association.

9. Daly A, Barry B, Gillespie S, Kulkarnie K, Richardson M. 1995. *Carbohydrate Counting: Moving On.* Alexandria, VA: American Diabetes Association; Chicago, IL: The American Dietetic Association.

10. Daly A, Barry B, Gillespie S, Kulkarnie K, Richardson M. 1995. *Carbohydrate Counting: Using Carbohydrate/Insulin Ratios.* Alexandria, VA: American Diabetes Association; Chicago, IL: The American Dietetic Association.

11. Paige MS, Heins JM. 1993. Nutritional management of diabetic patients during intensive insulin therapy. *Diabetes Educator* 14(6):505–509.

12. American Diabetes Association. 1997. Position statement: Diabetes mellitus and exercise. *Diabetes Care* 20(12):1908–1912.

EATING DISORDERS

Eating disorders range from unhealthy dieting and preoccupation with body size to life-threatening disorders (e.g., anorexia nervosa, bulimia nervosa) that merit inclusion in the *Diagnostic and Statistical Manual of Mental Disorders* (DSM-IV).[1,2] In between are eating-related behaviors, attitudes, and psychopathologies that vary in frequency and severity.

The DSM-IV criteria for anorexia nervosa, bulimia nervosa, and eating disorders not otherwise specified follow on pages 191 and 192.

Significance

Eating disorders have been observed in both sexes and across socioeconomic and racial/ethnic groups. The prevalence of anorexia nervosa and bulimia nervosa is thought to be 1 to 2 percent among adolescent females. With anorexia nervosa, estimates of mortality rates from all causes vary greatly, averaging 5 to 8 percent, with some as high as 20 percent.[3,4] Death may be due to cardiac arrhythmia, acute cardiovascular failure, gastric hemorrhaging, or suicide. The major medical complications seen include the following:[5]

Cardiac arrhythmia

Dehydration and electrolyte imbalances

Delayed growth and development

Endocrinological disturbances (e.g., menstrual dysfunction, hypothermia)

Gastrointestinal problems

Oral health problems (e.g., enamel demineralization, salivary dysfunction)

Osteopenia, osteoporosis

Protein/calorie malnutrition and its consequences

Nutritional Adequacy and Medical Complications

The actual food intake of children and adolescents with eating disorders varies considerably and is difficult to assess. Food intake is greatly influenced by food avoidance, the duration of restrictive eating episodes, the presence of binge eating, and other factors. Generally, specific vitamin and mineral deficiencies are not present; however, it must be emphasized that supplements are not a substitute for a healthy balanced diet.

Following are the nutrition inadequacies commonly seen in children and adolescents with eating disorders:

- *Energy.* Low energy intake, sometimes less than 500 calories per day, is a hallmark of anorexia nervosa.

- *Protein.* Protein intake is often low enough to result in clinical signs of protein deficiency in children and adolescents with restrictive types of eating disorders. Meat, poultry, fish, eggs, and dairy products are good sources of protein that are sometimes avoided by children and adolescents with eating disorders.

- *Calcium.* Because children and adolescents with eating disorders typically have insufficient dietary calcium intake, which can cause bone mineral loss, it is essential to maximize intake of

Diagnostic Criteria for 307.1 Anorexia Nervosa

A. Refusal to maintain body weight at or above a minimally normal weight for age and height (e.g., weight loss leading to maintenance of body weight less than 85% of that expected; or failure to make expected weight gain during period of growth, leading to body weight less than 85% of that expected).

B. Intense fear of gaining weight or becoming fat, even though underweight.

C. Disturbance in the way in which one's body weight or shape is experienced, undue influence of body weight or shape on self-evaluation, or denial of the seriousness of the current low body weight.

D. In postmenarcheal females, amenorrhea, i.e., the absence of at least three consecutive menstrual cycles. (A woman is considered to have amenorrhea if her periods occur only following hormone, e.g., estrogen, administration.)

Specify type:

Restricting Type: During the current episode of Anorexia Nervosa, the person has not regularly engaged in binge-eating or purging behavior (i.e., self-induced vomiting or the misuse of laxatives, diuretics, or enemas).

Binge-Eating/Purging Type: During the current episode of Anorexia Nervosa, the person has regularly engaged in binge-eating or purging behaviors (i.e., self-induced vomiting or the misuse of laxatives, diuretics, or enemas).

Diagnostic Criteria for 307.51 Bulimia Nervosa

A. Recurrent episodes of binge eating. An episode of binge eating is characterized by both of the following:
   (1) eating, in a discrete period of time (e.g., within any 2-hour period), an amount of food that is definitely larger than most people would eat during a similar period of time and under similar circumstances
   (2) a sense of lack of control over eating during the episode (e.g., a feeling that one cannot stop eating or control what or how much one is eating)

B. Recurrent, inappropriate compensatory behavior in order to prevent weight gain, such as self-induced vomiting; misuse of laxatives, diuretics, enemas, or other medications; fasting; or excessive exercise.

C. The binge eating and inappropriate compensatory behaviors both occur, on average, at least twice a week for 3 months.

D. Self-evaluation is unduly influenced by body shape and weight.

E. The disturbance does not occur exclusively during episodes of Anorexia Nervosa.

Specify type:

Purging Type: During the current episode of Bulimia Nervosa, the person has regularly engaged in self-induced vomiting or the misuse of laxatives, diuretics, or enemas.

Nonpurging Type: During the current episode of Bulimia Nervosa, the person has used other inappropriate compensatory behaviors, such as fasting or excessive exercise, but has not regularly engaged in self-induced vomiting or the misuse of laxatives, diuretics, or enemas.

Diagnostic Criteria for 307.50 Eating Disorder Not Otherwise Specified

The Eating Disorder Not Otherwise Specified category is for disorders of eating that do not meet the criteria for any specific eating disorder. Examples include

1. For females, all of the criteria for Anorexia Nervosa are met except the individual has regular menses.

2. All of the criteria for Anorexia Nervosa are met except that, despite significant weight loss, the individual's current weight is in the normal range.

3. All of the criteria for Bulimia Nervosa are met except that the binge-eating and inappropriate compensatory mechanisms occur at a frequency of less than twice a week or for a duration of less than 3 months.

4. The regular use of inappropriate compensatory behavior by an individual of normal body weight after eating small amounts of food (e.g., self-induced vomiting after the consumption of two cookies).

5. Repeatedly chewing and spitting out, but not swallowing, large amounts of food.

6. Binge-eating disorder: recurrent episodes of binge-eating in the absence of the regular use of inappropriate compensatory behaviors characteristic of Bulimia Nervosa.

Source: Reprinted, with permission, from the American Psychiatric Association.[2(p544–550)] © 1994, American Psychiatric Association.

milk, yogurt, and other dairy products, and to use calcium supplements if needed.

- *Zinc.* When protein intake is low, zinc intake is usually limited as well. It is especially important to promote zinc- and protein-rich foods (e.g., milk, meat, whole grains) because of zinc's role in taste dysfunction and appetite.

- *Vitamin B_{12}.* Intake of vitamin B_{12} may be a concern only in those with restrictive eating practices who are also strict vegetarians and who may not consume enough dairy products or eggs to obtain the RDA of vitamin B_{12}.

Screening and Assessment

Early identification of children and adolescents with eating disorders has been linked to better long-term outcomes. However, it can be difficult to identify children and adolescents who have eating disorders or who are at high risk for developing such disorders because they may avoid medical visits; present with gastrointestinal complaints, amenorrhea, or sports injuries; or seek assistance with weight loss. Parents sometimes seek medical help for their children or adolescents because of concerns about unexplained weight loss or suspicion of self-induced vomiting.

Screening

Eating disorder screening, which can be incorporated into any health visit, includes many components of an annual physical or sports checkup. In addition to conducting the physical examination (including determination of body mass index [BMI]), the health professional should talk with the child or adolescent to obtain information about body image and weight history, eating behaviors and meal patterns, physical activity, and health

Table 14. Screening Elements and Warning Signs for Individuals with Eating Disorders

Screening	Warning Signs
Body image and weight history	Distorted body image Extreme dissatisfaction with body shape or size Profound fear of gaining weight or becoming fat Unexplained weight change or fluctuations greater than 10 lb.
Eating and related behaviors	Very low caloric intake; avoidance of fatty foods Poor appetite; frequent bloating Difficulty eating in front of others Chronic dieting despite not being overweight Binge-eating episodes Self-induced vomiting; laxative or diuretic use
Meal patterns	Fasting or frequent meal-skipping to lose weight Erratic meal pattern with wide variations in caloric intake
Physical activity	Participation in physical activity with weight or size requirement (e.g., gymnastics, wrestling, ballet) Overtraining or "compulsive" attitude about physical activity
Psychosocial assessment	Depression Constant thoughts about food or weight Pressure from others to be a certain shape or size History of physical or sexual abuse or other traumatizing life event
Health history	Secondary amenorrhea or irregular menses Fainting episodes or frequent lightheadedness Constipation or diarrhea unexplained by other causes
Physical examination	BMI < 5th percentile Varying heart rate, decreased blood pressure after arising suddenly Hypothermia; cold intolerance Loss of muscle mass Tooth enamel demineralization

Sources: Perkins et al.,[7] Adams and Shafer,[8] and AMA.[9]

history, and should administer a brief psychosocial assessment. If any warning indicators of eating disorders are present (see Table 14), the health professional needs to evaluate further, with the use of assessments listed below.

However, the presence of a warning sign does not always indicate an eating disorder. Physically active children and adolescents may experience occasional gastrointestinal complaints, dizziness, irregular meal patterns, and menstrual irregularities without having an eating disorder. Consultation with health professionals experienced in eating disorders can help distinguish "typical" child or adolescent eating behaviors from a more serious eating disorder.[6]

Note that bulimia nervosa can also damage teeth. Vomiting exposes the teeth to acidic vomitus, which demineralizes the enamel and slowly dissolves the teeth. The health professional should refer an individual to a dentist if damage is apparent. With bulimia nervosa, enlargement of the parotid glands may also be present.

Assessment

If the child or adolescent is at high risk for an eating disorder (based on the indicators listed in Table 14), a number of assessments should be performed in addition to the initial screening. These assessments are best done by an interdisciplinary team of health specialists working together to evaluate the child or adolescent at high risk.

Medical History and Physical Assessment

■ Rule out organic illness as an explanation for weight loss or menstrual abnormalities.

■ Ask about history of binge eating and/or compensatory behaviors (e.g., self-induced vomiting; laxative, diuretic, or diet pill use; excessive physical activity). If the child or adolescent is diabetic with elevated HgbA$_{1c}$ levels, evaluate the possibility of insulin-withholding as a means of weight control.

■ Repeat assessment for orthostatic changes in pulse and blood pressure.

■ Assess the need for hospitalization[10] (see the Referral section below).

■ Laboratory tests are not definitive markers for diagnosing the presence of eating disorders; children and adolescents with eating disorders often have results within the normal range when screened with the following tests:

- *Amylase.* Pancreatic amylase (and sometimes blood) is elevated in some children or adolescents who are vomiting regularly.

- *Magnesium.* Hypomagnesemia (decreased magnesium in the blood) may be observed with laxative abuse.

- *Potassium.* Hypokalemia (decreased potassium in the blood) may be observed with prolonged malnutrition or with purging.

- *Urine ketones.* These compounds may be elevated because of chronic fasting or inadequate intake.

- *Urine specific gravity.* This measurement may be elevated (suggesting dehydration) or may be low because of excessive fluid intake.

- *Other tests.* Although liver function tests and thyroid tests may be abnormal, both will usually return to normal if the child or adolescent resumes eating healthy foods regularly.

Nutritional Assessment

■ Take a detailed weight history, including history of binge eating or purging (e.g., self-induced vomiting; laxative or diuretic use). Some children and adolescents do not want to talk about their eating and physical activity behaviors, and are more likely to answer health-focused questions phrased in a supportive, non-blaming way. (For example, "To make sure your body is getting everything it needs, I'm going to ask you a couple of questions about what you are eating and drinking. Can you tell me everything you had to eat or drink yesterday?")

■ Request a 3- or 5-day food/physical activity record that provides information on the specific types and quantities of food consumed, as well as the places and times food was eaten, the number of other people present, and the types of physical activities performed during the time period.

■ Assess triceps skinfold and arm-muscle circumference for estimate of body fat stores and muscle mass depletion.

■ Rule out clinical nutrition deficiencies as causes of symptoms such as hair loss or dry skin.

Psychiatric/Psychological Assessment

■ Interview the child or adolescent and the parents about circumstances surrounding the onset of changes in eating behavior or weight.[11]

■ Assess for depression, and rule out other psychiatric disorders (e.g., anxiety disorder, obsessive-compulsive disorder, bipolar disorder) as primary or comorbid conditions that might explain changes in eating behavior and preoccupation with body weight and shape.[11]

■ Assess risk of suicide.[11]

Referral and Management

Comprehensive assessment and treatment require an interdisciplinary team that has experience in treating eating disorders in children or adolescents and that can provide nutrition counseling, medical care and monitoring, psychiatric evaluation, and individual and/or family therapy. Referral to an eating disorder treatment program should be considered if an interdisciplinary team is not available or if hospitalization is indicated.

Hospitalization may be needed if the child or adolescent is severely malnourished, shows metabolic disturbances, or is at risk for suicide.[10] If the child or adolescent has anorexia nervosa, it is essential to ensure a gradual and carefully planned return to normal eating to prevent the "refeeding syndrome" associated with hypophosphatemia. Close monitoring of food intake and output, fluid status, physical activity, and body weight is necessary to accurately adjust the dietary recommendations for steady weight gain.

At minimum, children and adolescents with eating disorders need to be evaluated and followed long-term by a physician, a mental health professional (including at least one evaluation by a psychiatrist), and a dietitian. Because of the complexity of these disorders and the need to set clear, consistent behavioral limits, teamwork is essential.

Nutrition Counseling

The main goals in counseling children and adolescents with eating disorders are to enable them to achieve and maintain a BMI within the normal range (between the 15th and 85th percentiles), function well at school or work, and resume healthy eating behaviors. Nutrition counseling needs to be individually tailored, and coordinated with the medical and psychiatric/psychological management of the child or adolescent. Following are four interim nutrition goals for children or adolescents who have eating disorders, with specific strategies dietitians can use to help them achieve these goals:

1. Improve and restore nutritional adequacy.

   Set guidelines for food intake, based on the number of servings of specific foods (not calories).

   Recommend taking a vitamin and mineral supplement daily.

   Encourage children and adolescents to select foods that meet daily nutrition needs.

2. Maintain body weight (avoid additional weight loss or large weight fluctuations).

   Challenge the child's or adolescent's body image, comparing it with appropriate body weights and shapes.

   Encourage the child or adolescent to avoid self-weighing.

   Dispel myths about how weight loss occurs and explain why bodies store fat and why some fat from food is essential.

3. Decrease the frequency of binge eating and compensatory behaviors.

   Encourage the child or adolescent to eat three scheduled meals and one or two snacks each day.

   Help the child or adolescent identify situations that may trigger binge eating (e.g., parties), and plan ways to manage these situations.

4. Seek support from the family.

   Discourage family members from making comments to the child or adolescent about appearance, weight, or eating behaviors.

   Ask parents to remove all diet products and books, diet foods, and diet pills from the home.

   Establish and maintain regular family meals.

   Health professionals can help prevent eating disorders by promoting a positive body image and healthy attitudes toward food and physical activity.

Infancy and Early Childhood

Parents are usually very aware of their young children's eating habits and may have concerns about their nutritional adequacy, their risk of obesity, or their avoidance of foods. Eating disorders are not evident during this time.

- Emphasize the wide range of normal body weights for infants and children, and reassure parents who mistakenly believe their infant or child is overweight.

- Discourage restricted eating regimens for healthy infants and children.

- Promote feeding relationships that let infants and children respond to hunger and satiety cues.

- Encourage families to eat meals together regularly. Discuss ways to keep mealtimes pleasurable and to minimize struggles around food.

- Encourage parents to emphasize regular physical activity and promote a positive body image.

- Discourage the use of food to manipulate behavior, either as punishment or as incentive.

Middle Childhood

The eating and physical activity behaviors of children ages 5 to 10 years are affected a great deal by their expanding social world, and parents may feel they do not have much influence during this time. Parents need to be reminded that family behaviors and attitudes still significantly shape children's behaviors, and children should be encouraged to have a positive attitude toward food and a positive body image. Although eating disorders are less common in middle childhood than in adolescence, attitudes about body shape and size are developing, and experimentation with dieting has been observed.

- Suggest that parents review the kinds of foods available at home, especially snack foods and foods packed in school lunches. Encourage a balance of healthy foods.

- Discourage meal skipping or other restrictive eating behaviors, and encourage families to eat meals together whenever possible, at least once a day.

- Instruct family members not to tease the child about body weight, shape, or physical appearance and to avoid unhealthy dieting themselves.

- For 8- to 10-year-olds, briefly outline the ways their bodies will be changing as they experience puberty.

- Encourage regular physical activity for both the child and the family, with an emphasis on activities that the child enjoys and that contribute to overall fitness (see the Healthy Eating and Physical Activity chapter).

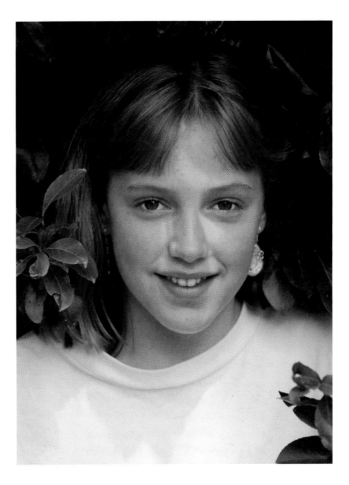

Adolescence

Puberty is the major physical hallmark of adolescence, with the normal biological changes sometimes viewed negatively by females (e.g., body fat deposits, menses) or more positively by males (e.g., greater height and muscle mass). Food and physical activity behaviors are often driven by the desire for physical attractiveness, by sports performance, and by friends' behaviors. Eating disorders develop most often during adolescence. Both adolescents and their families need nutrition counseling, but it is recommended that adolescents receive guidance individually.

- Describe pubertal changes, preferably before they occur, and be available as a "safe" person with whom adolescents can talk about body issues. With females, emphasize that body fat increases during this growth period; with males, discuss the wide variability in the timing of growth and maturation.

- Use BMI charts to assess an adolescent's relative weight, and discuss the broad range of weights considered normal for body shape and size.

- Discourage restrictive dieting or meal-skipping.

- Encourage regular but not excessive physical activity to maintain health and weight.

- Instruct family members to avoid teasing the adolescent about body weight, shape, or physical appearance and to avoid unhealthy dieting themselves.

- For overweight adolescents, carefully phrase recommendations for weight loss, and help them identify behaviors they can change.

References

1. Van der Ham T, Meulman JJ, Van Strien DC, Van Engeland H. 1997. Empirically based subgroupings of eating disorders in adolescents: A longitudinal perspective. *British Journal of Psychiatry* 170:363–368.

2. American Psychiatric Association. 1994. *Diagnostic and Statistical Manual of Mental Disorders* (4th ed.). Washington, DC: American Psychiatric Association.

3. Neumarker KJ. 1997. Mortality and sudden death in anorexia nervosa. *International Journal of Eating Disorders* 21(3):205–212.

4. Moller-Madsen S, Nystrup J, Nielsen S. 1996. Mortality in anorexia nervosa in Denmark during the period 1970–1987. *Acta Psychiatrica Scandinavica* 94(6): 454–459.

5. Hall RC, Beresford TP. 1989. Medical complications of anorexia and bulimia. *Psychiatric Medicine* 7(4): 165–185.

6. Emans SJ. Menarche and beyond—Do eating and exercise make a difference? 1997. *Pediatric Annals* 26 (supplement):S137–S141.

7. Perkins K, Ferrari N, Rosas A, Bessette R, Williams A, Omar H. 1997. You won't know unless you ask: The biopsychosocial interview for adolescents. *Clinical Pediatrics* 36(2):79–86.

8. Adams LB, Shafer MB. 1988. Early manifestations of eating disorders in adolescents: Defining those at risk. *Journal of Nutrition Education* 20:307–313.

9. American Medical Association, Department of Adolescent Health. 1995. *Guidelines for Adolescent Preventive Services (GAPS): Recommendations Monograph* (2nd ed.). Chicago, IL: American Medical Association, Department of Adolescent Health.

10. Kreipe RE, Higgins LA. 1996. Anorexia nervosa. In Rickert VI, ed., *Adolescent Nutrition: Assessment and Management* (pp. 159–180). New York, NY: Chapman and Hall (Aspen Publishers).

11. American Psychiatric Association. 1993. Practice guideline for eating disorders. *American Journal of Psychiatry* 150(2):212–228.

Suggested Reading

Fisher M, Golden NH, Katzman DK, Kreipe RE, Rees J, Schebendach J, Sigman G, Ammerman S, Hobermann HM. 1995. Eating disorders in adolescents: A background paper. *Journal of Adolescent Health* 16(6):420–437.

Katzman DK, Zipursky RB. 1997. Adolescents with anorexia nervosa: The impact of the disorder on bones and brain. *Annals of the New York Academy of Sciences* 817:127–137.

Kreipe RE, Golden NH, Katzman DK, Fisher M, Rees J, Tonkin RS, Silber TJ, Sigman G, Schebendach J, Ammerman SD. 1995. Eating disorder in adolescents. A position of the Society for Adolescent Medicine. *Journal of Adolescent Health* 16(6):476–479.

Position of The American Dietetic Association: Nutrition intervention in the treatment of anorexia nervosa, bulimia nervosa, and binge eating. 1994. *Journal of The American Dietetic Association* 94(8):902–907.

Schebendach J, Nussbaum MP. 1992. Nutrition management in adolescents with eating disorders. *Adolescent Medicine: State of the Art Review* 3:541–548.

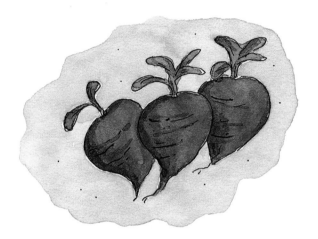

OBESITY

Obesity is defined as the presence of excess adipose (fatty) tissue in the body. The term "overweight" may connote a milder degree of excess fat than "obesity," but there are no clearly defined criteria to distinguish between the two terms. Thus, the two are used interchangeably.[1]

Although the underlying causes are not fully understood, obesity is a complex chronic disease involving genetics, metabolism, and physiology, as well as environmental and psychosocial factors. Inappropriate eating behaviors and low levels of physical activity are contributing to the continuing rise in the prevalence of obesity among children and adolescents.[2]

Significance

Obesity is a major public health problem. Studies over the past 2 decades have shown a dramatic increase in the prevalence of obesity among children (including those younger than 5 years of age) and adolescents.[3,4] Recent data from the National Center for Health Statistics (NCHS) indicate that more than 1 in 5 U.S. children and adolescents are overweight.[3]

Few studies have examined the long-term effect of child or adolescent obesity on adult morbidity and mortality. Longitudinal studies of children followed into young adulthood suggest that overweight children may become overweight adults, particularly if obesity is present in adolescence.[5-7] Overweight in adolescence is associated with current levels of and changes in blood pressure, blood lipids, lipoproteins, and insulin.[8] Perhaps the most widespread consequences of childhood obesity are psychosocial, including discrimination.[8,9]

Health professionals should be aware of the demographic and personal risk factors for childhood and adolescent obesity, and they should be diligent in prevention strategies and screening.[2] Children and adolescents are considered at high risk for overweight if (1) one or both of their parents are overweight, (2) they live in families with low incomes, (3) they have chronic illness or disabilities that limit mobility, or (4) they are members of certain racial/ethnic minority groups (preadolescent and adolescent African-American females; Hispanic populations; and American Indian/Alaska Native populations).[2,4] Norms for a "healthy" appearance may vary across cultures; children, adolescents, and their families should be counseled within a cultural context.

Prevention

Enough is known to guide efforts to reverse the trend of increasing obesity.[2] Because obesity is difficult to treat, efforts should focus on prevention. Although genetic influences largely determine whether a person may become overweight, environmental influences (e.g., eating behaviors, physical inactivity) may determine the manifestation and extent of the obesity.

The most important strategies for preventing obesity are healthy eating behaviors, regular physical activity, and reduced sedentary activity (e.g., watching television and videotapes, playing computer games). These preventive strategies are part of a healthy lifestyle that should be developed during early childhood. The goal is to teach and model healthy and positive attitudes toward food and physical activity without emphasizing body weight. Behavioral techniques are needed to encourage healthy eating and physical activity behaviors.

Healthy Eating

Parents need information on how to encourage their child to eat in a healthy manner, beginning when the child is very young.[2] Suggestions include limiting the duration of bottlefeeding; ensuring appropriate use of low-fat and nonfat milk after 2 years of age; limiting consumption of high-sugar foods (including juices); being aware of portion sizes of foods, especially high-fat and high-sugar foods; limiting the frequency of fast-food meals; and encouraging family members to drink water.

Achieving a modest reduction of fat in the family diet is a good way to prevent excess weight gain. Fat should not be restricted in children younger than 2 years of age; children older than 2 should gradually adopt eating practices so that by age 5 their fat intake is no more than 30 percent of their total calories.[10] The Dietary Guidelines for Americans provide an eating guide for healthy persons ages 2 years and older. (See the Healthy Eating and Physical Activity chapter.)

Physical Activity

Physical activity (approximately 30 minutes) on most, if not all, days of the week is beneficial for people of all ages.[11] Health professionals routinely need to discuss physical activity practices with family members and to help them develop ways to increase physical activity and decrease sedentary activity in their lives. Solutions might include playfully chasing young children around the yard or playground, dancing to music before dinner, or riding a station-ary bike while watching television.[2] Involving children and adolescents in team sports can help build skill levels and self-confidence, foster teamwork, and increase energy expenditures.

Screening

Body mass index (BMI) is recommended for screening children and adolescents. BMI is easily calculated from weight and height measures (kg/m^2) and can be plotted on a standard growth chart (e.g., the revised Centers for Disease Control and Prevention [CDC]/National Center for Health Statistics [NCHS] growth chart). BMI reflects body mass rather than body fat, but correlates with measures of subcutaneous and total body fat in children and adolescents. Some children and adolescents may have a high BMI because of a large, lean body mass from physical activity, high muscularity, or frame size. An elevated triceps skinfold (above the 95th percentile on the standard CDC/NCHS growth chart) can confirm excess body fat in children or adolescents.[1]

The following screening guidelines are based on the recommendations of an expert committee of pediatric health professionals.[1]

- Children older than 2 and adolescents with BMIs at or above the 95th percentile for age and sex are considered overweight and should receive an in-depth assessment.

- Children older than 2 and adolescents with BMIs between the 85th and 95th percentiles for age and sex are considered at risk for becoming overweight and should be screened and evaluated carefully, with particular attention to family history and secondary complications of obesity, including hypertension and dyslipidemias.

Figure 5. Recommended Overweight Screening Procedures

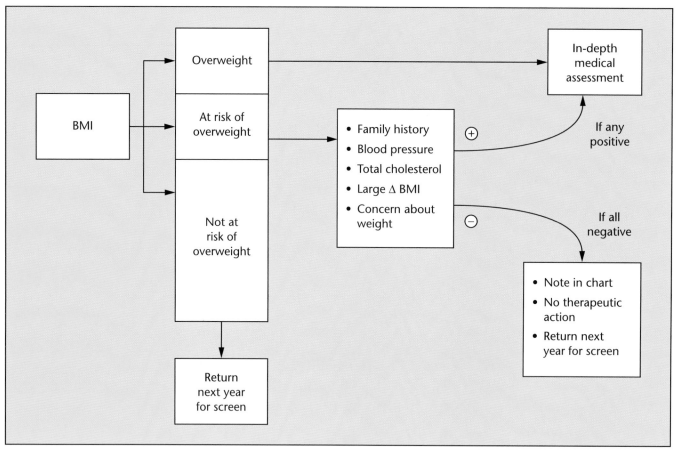

Source: Reproduced, with permission, from Figure 1, Himes and Dietz.[12(p312)] ©1994, *American Journal of Clinical Nutrition,* American Society for Clinical Nutrition.

- Children (older than 2) and adolescents with an annual increase of 3 to 4 BMI units should be evaluated.

Assessment

In-depth assessments (see Figure 5) are required to identify those children and adolescents with positive screens who are truly obese, to diagnose any underlying causes, and to provide a basis for a treatment plan.

Medical History

A thorough medical history must be conducted to identify any underlying syndromes or secondary complications.

Family History[7]

To identify familial risks for obesity, a family history is needed. This should include the presence of obesity, eating disorders, type 2 diabetes mellitus, cardiovascular disease, hypertension, dyslipidemia, and gallbladder disease in siblings, parents, aunts, uncles, or grandparents.

Dietary History

An assessment of the child's or adolescent's eating practices (quantity, quality, and timing) will identify both foods and patterns of eating that may lead to excessive caloric intake. If the health professional's dietary assessment skills are limited, a dietitian should obtain the dietary history.

Physical Activity History

A careful history of physical activity is needed to quantify activity levels as well as time spent in sedentary behaviors. Any history of medical contraindications to physical activity should be noted (e.g., asthma, joint disease).

Physical Examination

The physical examination will provide information about the degree of overweight and any potential underlying syndromes or complications of obesity. Height, weight, and BMI should be plotted on a standard growth chart (e.g., the revised CDC/NCHS growth chart) to identify the degree of overweight.

Laboratory Testing

Degree of overweight, family history, and the physical examination will guide the choice of laboratory tests.

Psychological Evaluation

Readiness to change. A weight-management program for children, adolescents, or their families who are not ready to change may be both ineffective and harmful because it can affect the child's or adoles-

cent's self-esteem and impair future weight-loss efforts. A practical way to address readiness is to ask members of the family how concerned they are about a family member's weight, whether they believe weight loss is possible, and what practices need to be changed. Assess family readiness with questions such as "How concerned are you about this problem?" "Have you thought about or tried to lose weight? If so, what did you try, and when did you try it?" In families with younger children, the parent who is ready to change can successfully modify the family diet and physical activity. Therapeutic efforts should focus on those families that are concerned about their child's weight and ready to make changes.

Families who are not ready to change may express a lack of concern about the child's or adolescent's obesity, may believe that obesity is inevitable and cannot be changed, or may lack interest in modifying eating practices or physical activities. Unless a serious complication of obesity already exists, families that are not ready to change should be given information about the health consequences of obesity and told that help is available when they are ready. Health professionals should continue to foster a positive relationship with the family so that treatment may be possible in the future.

Eating disorders. Children or adolescents who feel unable to control their consumption of large amounts of food or who report vomiting or use of laxatives to avoid weight gain may have an eating disorder. In this situation, the child or adolescent should be referred to an eating disorder program that incorporates psychological assessment/treatment, medical assessment/treatment, and nutrition counseling.

Figure 6. Recommendations for Weight Goals

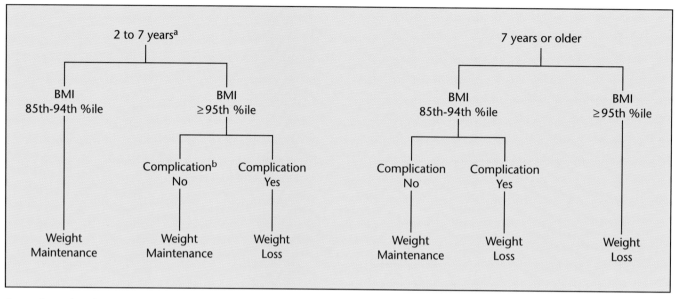

Source: Reproduced, with permission, from Figure 2, Barlow and Dietz.[1] Copyright © 1998 American Academy of Pediatrics.

[a] Indicates that children younger than 2 years should be referred to a pediatric obesity center for treatment.

[b] Indicates complications such as mild hypertension, dyslipidemias, and insulin resistance. Patients with acute complications, such as pseudotumor cerebri, sleep apnea, obesity hypoventilation syndrome, or orthopedic problems, should be referred to a pediatric obesity center.

Depression. Overweight children or adolescents who are depressed may exhibit sleep disturbance, hopelessness and sadness, and appetite changes. As with eating disorders, depression in children or adolescents requires psychological evaluation and treatment.

Treatment

The primary goal of a program to treat uncomplicated obesity is to achieve healthy eating and physical activity behaviors, rather than obtaining ideal body weight. Treatment programs need to emphasize the skills necessary to change behaviors and to maintain those changes. The first step toward weight control for all overweight children (older than 2 years) and adolescents is weight main-

tenance, which can be achieved by modest changes in food intake and physical activity. Children and adolescents who are excessively overweight (weighing 180 percent or more of their ideal body weight) cannot be expected to increase activity levels dramatically. Small incremental changes should be the goal.

Weight loss, if warranted, should be only about 1 pound per month.[1] Recommendations for achieving weight goals are shown in Figure 6. An appropriate weight goal for all obese children and adolescents is a BMI at or below the 85th percentile, although such a goal should be secondary to the primary goal of healthy eating, regular physical activity, and psychological well-being.

Approaches to Treatment

Children and adolescents receiving anticipatory guidance or treatment for obesity need to be monitored carefully by health professionals from a variety of disciplines, which can help families achieve many aspects of a weight-management program. Experience in cognitive-behavioral approaches to intervention are helpful. The following approaches are based on the recommendations of an expert committee of pediatric health professionals.[1]

- Intervention should begin early.

- The approach should involve family members. The goal is to help family members achieve healthy behaviors rather than to single out the overweight child or adolescent.

- Start slowly. Ask families to suggest one or two changes, then help them determine how to monitor the changes.

- Families should learn how to monitor eating and physical activity as part of the treatment process.

- Because weight maintenance is an important first step, families of children or adolescents who have maintained their weight should be praised for their success.

- Treatment programs should seek to institute permanent changes, avoiding short-term diets or physical activity programs aimed at rapid weight loss.

- Health professionals need to encourage and empathize rather than criticize.

- Health professionals need to educate families about the medical complications of obesity.

- Children and adolescents should never be placed on a restricted diet to lose weight except for medical reasons, when closely supervised by a health professional.

Parenting Skills

Families can benefit from guidance on effective behavioral management and limit-setting. Parents need support and guidance in the skills required to help prevent or treat child or adolescent obesity. Health professionals can help support parents by emphasizing the following principles:[1]

- Find reasons to praise the child's or adolescent's behavior.

- Never use food as a reward. Plan activities and special times together to reward desired behavior.

- Be consistent.

- Establish daily times for family meals and snacks.

- Determine what types of foods are offered at what times, and allow the child or adolescent to decide whether to eat.

- Allow children developmentally appropriate control of food.

- Offer healthy food options.

- Model healthy eating and physical activity behaviors.

- Encourage regular physical activity, and make it fun.

- Limit the amount of time spent watching television and videotapes and playing computer games to 1 to 2 hours per day. Focus on ways to make television viewing more difficult.

- Assist the child or adolescent in dealing with teasing or hurtful social situations resulting from overweight.

Referral

Children or adolescents who present with serious complications of obesity need to be closely monitored by a health professional and referred (if possible) to a pediatric obesity treatment program. Complications that indicate referral or consultation include pseudotumor cerebri, sleep apnea, obesity hypoventilation syndrome, Blount's disease (tibia vara), slipped capital femoral epiphysis, and severe overweight (above the 99th percentile).[1]

References

1. Barlow SE, Dietz WH. 1998. Obesity evaluation and treatment: Expert committee recommendations. In *Pediatrics Electronic Pages* 102(3):e29 [online journal]. Cited August 19, 1999; available from http://www.pediatrics.org/cgi/content/full/102/3/e29.

2. Christoffel KK, Ariza A. 1998. The epidemiology of overweight in children: Relevance for clinical care. *Pediatrics* 101(1):103–105.

3. Troiano RP, Flegal KM, Kuczmarski RJ, Campbell SM, Johnson CL. 1995. Overweight prevalence and trends for children and adolescents. The National Health and Nutrition Examination Surveys, 1963 to 1991. *Archives of Pediatrics and Adolescent Medicine* 149(10):1085–1091.

4. Troiano RP, Flegal KM. 1998. Overweight children and adolescents: Description, epidemiology, and demographics. *Pediatrics* 101(3, Part 2):497–504.

5. Serdula MK, Ivery D, Coates RJ, Freedman DS, Williamson DF, Byers T. 1993. Do obese children become obese adults? A review of the literature. *Preventive Medicine* 22(2):167–177.

6. Guo SS, Roche AF, Chumlea WC, Gardner JD, Siervogel RM. 1994. The predictive value of childhood body mass index values for overweight at age 35 y. *American Journal of Clinical Nutrition* 59(4):810–819.

7. Braddon FE, Rodgers B, Wadsworth ME, Davies JM. 1986. Onset of obesity in a 36 year birth cohort study. *British Medical Journal (Clinical Research Edition)* 293(6542):299–303.

8. Gidding SS, Leibel RL, Daniels S, Rosenbaum M, Van Horn L, Marx GR. 1996. Understanding obesity in youth. A statement for healthcare professionals from the Committee on Atherosclerosis and Hypertension in the Young of the Council on Cardiovascular Disease in the Young and the Nutrition Committee, American Heart Association. Writing Group. *Circulation* 94(12):3383–3387.

9. Dietz WH. 1998. Health consequences of obesity in youth: Childhood predictors of adult disease. *Pediatrics* 101(3, Part 2):518–525.

10. U.S. Department of Agriculture and U.S. Department of Health and Human Services. 1995. *Nutrition and Your Health: Dietary Guidelines for Americans* (4th ed.). Hyattsville, MD: U.S. Department of Agriculture.

11. Centers for Disease Control and Prevention, National Center for Chronic Disease Prevention and Health Promotion, President's Council on Physical Fitness and Sports. 1996. *Physical Activity and Health: A Report of the Surgeon General*. Washington, DC: Centers for Disease Control and Prevention, National Center for Chronic Disease Prevention and Health Promotion.

12. Himes JH, Dietz WH. 1994. Guidelines for overweight in adolescent preventive services: Recommendations from an expert committee. *American Journal of Clinical Nutrition* 59:307–316.

HYPERLIPIDEMIA

Hyperlipidemia or hyperlipoproteinemia typically refers to any elevation of blood lipid levels (e.g., total cholesterol, triglycerides, or lipoproteins).[1] Although terms such as hypercholesterolemia are often used interchangeably with hyperlipidemia, there are subtle differences. Hypercholesterolemia refers to excess blood cholesterol. Dyslipoproteinemia or dyslipidemia describes abnormal levels of blood lipoproteins (e.g., low levels of high-density lipoproteins [HDLs], elevated low-density or very-low-density lipoproteins [LDLs or VLDLs]). Table 15 lists the range of acceptable, borderline, and high cholesterol levels for at-risk children and adolescents.

Significance

At least one-quarter of children and adolescents are estimated to have borderline-high or high cholesterol levels.[2] In adults, elevated blood-cholesterol levels are strongly associated with atherosclerosis (hardening of the arteries) and death from coronary heart disease (CHD).[3] The process of atherosclerosis begins in childhood, with the appearance of fatty streaks in the arteries. Dietary interventions may lower total and LDL cholesterol levels and should be the initial therapy for hyperlipidemia.[1]

Prevention

The following dietary recommendations have been issued for the prevention of atherosclerosis in children 2 years of age and older:[4(pp412–414),5]

- Children younger than 2 years of age should not have their fat or dietary cholesterol intake restricted because of the high energy required during this time of rapid growth and development.

- Children 1 year of age and older should eat a variety of foods to ensure adequate nutrition. At age 2, children gradually need to begin eating fewer high-fat foods, so that by age 5, they receive no more than 30 percent of their calories from fat.

- Children should be encouraged to maintain or increase their levels of regular physical activity.

- Older children and adolescents need to be counseled on the consequences of tobacco use and provided with strategies for avoiding it.

To promote lower cholesterol levels in all healthy children and adolescents ages 2 to 18, the following pattern of nutrient intake is recommended:[5]

- Saturated fat should be less than 10 percent of the total number of calories consumed.

- Over several days, total fat should be between 20 and 30 percent of total calories.

- Dietary cholesterol should be no more than 300 mg per day.

Screening

Early identification and treatment of children and adolescents with elevated lipid levels may reduce their risk of developing premature CHD. A family history of premature cardiovascular disease and/or high blood cholesterol are the most significant risk indicators for screening lipid levels in chil-

Table 15. Classification of Cholesterol Levels in High-Risk Children and Adolescents[a]

	Total Cholesterol, mg/dL	LDL Cholesterol, mg/dL
Acceptable	<170	< 110
Borderline	170–199	110–129
High	≥ 200	≥ 130

Source: Reproduced from the National Cholesterol Education Program.[1(p43)]
[a]I.e., children and adolescents from families with hypercholesterolemia or premature cardiovascular disease.

dren and adolescents. Health professionals need to identify children and adolescents at highest risk for developing accelerated atherosclerosis by screening cholesterol levels in those who meet any of the following criteria:[5(pp143–144)]

- A parent or grandparent (≤ 55 years of age) who has been diagnosed with coronary artherosclerosis (on the basis of a coronary arteriography), including those who have undergone balloon angioplasty or coronary artery bypass surgery

- A parent or grandparent (≤ 55 years of age) with documented myocardial infarction, angina pectoris, peripheral vascular disease, cerebrovascular disease, or sudden cardiac death

- A parent with a high blood cholesterol level (≥ 240 mg/dL)

Children and adolescents whose family history cannot be reliably obtained—particularly those with other risk factors—should also be screened to determine their need for medical and nutrition guidance.[5(p144)]

Other risk factors that contribute to early onset of CHD include the following:[5]

- Family history of premature CHD, cerebrovascular disease, or occlusive peripheral vascular disease

- Cigarette smoking

- Elevated blood pressure

- Low HDL cholesterol concentrations (< 35 mg/dL)

- Severe obesity (BMI ≥ 95th percentile)

- Diabetes mellitus

- Physical inactivity

Medical Screening

- Evaluate for and treat secondary causes of hyperlipidemia (e.g., corticosteroids, anabolic steroids, certain oral contraceptives, Accutane, anorexia nervosa, hypothyroidism, diabetes mellitus, pregnancy).[6,7]

- Evaluate for familial lipid disorder and clinical signs of hyperlipidemia.[6,7]

- Identify other risk factors.[6,7]

- Screen all family members.[6,7]

Nutrition Screening

- Interview the child or adolescent and the parent(s) to assess food purchasing and preparation habits as well as eating patterns. Provide nutrition counseling.[7,8]

- Ask the child or adolescent to complete a 3-day food record to supplement the dietary interview. (If the child is younger than 10, the parent should complete the food record.)[7,8]

Monitoring

Children and adolescents with hyperlipidemia need to have their blood cholesterol, eating behaviors, and other risk factors monitored regularly. Those with borderline elevations in blood cholesterol should be rechecked within 1 year, but those with higher LDLs or higher total cholesterol values should be seen 1 to 2 months after initial nutrition counseling to reevaluate their status. Three-day food records can be collected at least twice a year to help assess progress. If blood lipid levels have not improved or dietary goals have not been achieved, more intensive instruction may be required. With familial lipid disorders, blood lipid levels may not improve appreciably, even with excellent adherence to a regimen. This may be an appropriate time for referral to a lipid center and/or consideration of drug therapy.

Nutrition Counseling

Following are the major components of nutrition counseling for children and adolescents with hyperlipidemia.

- Seek support from the child's or adolescent's family.
- Explain and encourage adherence to the National Cholesterol Education Program dietary guidelines.[1]
- Ensure the nutritional adequacy of the child's or adolescent's diet.
- Teach skills for appropriately selecting and preparing food.
- Help the child or adolescent and the family plan ahead for special occasions and provide flexibility in food choices.

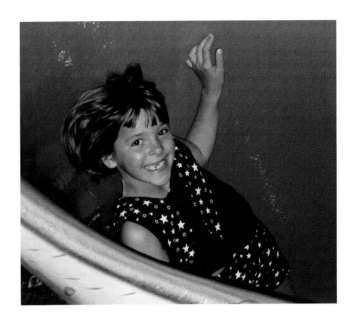

- Encourage the reduction of other CHD risk factors.
- Encourage regular physical activity and sound approaches to weight management. If the child or adolescent is overweight, encourage daily physical activity.

Following are age-appropriate strategies for preventing or treating hyperlipidemia.

Infancy and Early Childhood

When infants are introduced to cow's milk at about 1 year, whole milk should be given because of the child's need for higher levels of fat. Children older than 2 years can be given 2-percent, low-fat, or skim milk.

Serving three healthy meals plus three snacks each day is the best way to satisfy the young child's appetite.

Middle Childhood

The dietary recommendations of the National Cholesterol Education Program and the American Academy of Pediatrics are more than adequate to support growth in middle childhood, as long as meals are not skipped and snacks are available.[1,5] It is important to determine that foods are not being eliminated because of the child's refusal to try a lower-fat item. (For example, a child may drink less milk because of refusing to try a lower-fat milk). Gradually introducing the lower-fat milk (e.g., mixing equal portions of the higher-fat milk and the lower-fat milk for a week) or using it first in milkshakes may encourage acceptance.

During middle childhood, it is more difficult to monitor and control the food intake of a child with hyperlipidemia because of additional eating opportunities (e.g., at school, friends' houses, the movies, fast-food and other restaurants, and the neighborhood store). The health professional needs to weigh both the severity of the hyperlipidemia and the risk of developing CHD against the child's feelings of being deprived of favorite foods, and to build as much flexibility as possible into the child's diet.[1,7]

Adolescence

The National Cholesterol Education Program's dietary recommendations for adolescents with hyperlipidemia are nutritionally adequate, even during the rapid growth and development associated with puberty.[1] The need for flexibility in the diet is even greater for the adolescent with hyperlipidemia, who is eating away from home more frequently and assuming greater responsibility for selecting and preparing foods. Because elevated lipid levels are not associated with any pain or visible signs, it is challenging for adolescents to resist favorite foods to prevent health consequences far in the future. Consistent support from the family and health professionals for the adolescent's food choices is important in order to continue and reinforce dietary change. Adolescents in foster homes or halfway houses may face additional obstacles in trying to maintain a healthy, low-fat diet.[6,7,9]

Health professionals need to weigh the severity of the adolescent's hyperlipidemia against the relative risk that the adolescent may develop an eating disorder. The appropriate management of hyperlipidemia requires considerable attention to the fat content of foods, yet focusing on dietary or body fat is usually avoided in the prevention and treatment of eating disorders. Many adolescents with eating disorders initially justify their restrictive eating as an attempt to "eat healthy," denying they are trying to lose weight. In addition, secondary causes of hyperlipidemia include the metabolic changes seen in anorexia nervosa or the use of anabolic steroids for enhanced muscle mass. It may be useful to briefly screen for eating disorders in adolescents with hyperlipidemia.

Referral

Referral to a specialized lipid center should be considered for children and adolescents with a significant family history of premature heart disease or familial lipid disorders. Comprehensive nutrition counseling for the family is needed to help the child or adolescent adhere to the diet. Children and adolescents with LDL cholesterol higher than 130 mg/dL should be referred to a dietitian, who can tailor the diet to meet individual needs.

References

1. National Institutes of Health, National Heart, Lung, and Blood Institute, National Cholesterol Education Program. 1991. *Report of the Expert Panel on Blood Cholesterol Levels in Children and Adolescents.* Bethesda, MD: National Institutes of Health, National Heart, Lung, and Blood Institute, National Cholesterol Education Program.

2. Williams CL, Bollella M. 1995. Guidelines for screening, evaluating, and treating children with hypercholesterolemia. *Journal of Pediatric Health Care* 9(4):153–162.

3. Levine GN, Keaney JF Jr, Vita JA. 1995. Cholesterol reduction in cardiovascular disease. Clinical benefits and possible mechanisms. *The New England Journal of Medicine* 332(8):512–521.

4. American Academy of Pediatrics, Committee on Nutrition. 1998. *Pediatric Nutrition Handbook* (4th ed.). Elk Grove Village, IL: American Academy of Pediatrics.

5. American Academy of Pediatrics, Committee on Nutrition. 1998. Cholesterol in childhood. *Pediatrics* 101(1):141–147.

6. American Medical Association, Department of Adolescent Health. 1995. *Guidelines for Adolescent Preventive Services (GAPS): Recommendations Monograph* (2nd ed.). Chicago, IL: American Medical Association.

7. Arden MR, Schebendach JE. Disease prevention among youth: Atherosclerosis and hyperlipidemia. 1996. In Rickert VI, ed., *Adolescent Nutrition: Assessment and Management* (pp. 89–106). New York, NY: Chapman and Hall (Aspen Publishers).

8. Frank GC. 1988. Nutritional therapy for hyperlipidemia and obesity: Office treatment integrating the roles of the physician and the registered dietitian. *Journal of the American College of Cardiology* 12(4):1098–1101.

9. Kottke TE, Brekke ML, Solberg LI. 1993. Making "time" for preventive services. *Mayo Clinic Proceedings* 68(8):785–791.

HYPERTENSION

In children and adolescents, primary or essential hypertension is diagnosed when persistently elevated blood pressure cannot be explained by any underlying organic cause. According to the recommendations of the Task Force on Blood Pressure Control in Children, children and adolescents 1 to 17 years of age are considered hypertensive if their average systolic and/or diastolic blood pressure readings are at or above the 95th percentile (based on age, sex, and height) on at least three separate occasions.[1] Definitions of normal blood pressure and hypertension are as follows:

- Normal blood pressure: < 90th percentile

- High-normal blood pressure: ≥ 90th and < 95th percentiles

- Hypertension: ≥ 95th percentile (on three separate occasions)

In 1987 the Second Task Force on Blood Pressure Control in Children reported that children and adolescents with frequent blood pressure readings between the 90th and 95th percentiles for their age, sex, and height (unless tall for their age) are at risk for developing hypertension.[2] The task force advised that these children and adolescents with high-normal blood pressure should be followed regularly for early detection of further elevation in blood pressure. Tables 16 and 17 present the current blood pressure standards for the 90th and 95th percentiles for males and females ages 1 to 17 years, by percentile of height.[3]

For adolescents ages 18 and older, the severity of elevated blood pressure, when observed on two

or more occasions, is evaluated on the basis of the adult criteria in Table 18.[4]

Significance

Primary hypertension is an independent risk factor for cardiovascular disease. Familial patterns for primary hypertension have established that high blood pressure has its origins in childhood and adolescence; left untreated, high blood pressure generally will persist into adulthood. Primary hypertension is now considered the most common form

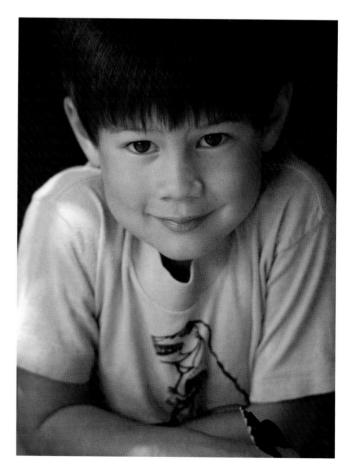

Table 16. Blood Pressure Levels for the 90th and 95th Percentiles of Blood Pressure for Boys Ages 1 to 17 Years

Age	BP Percentile[a]	Systolic BP (mm Hg), by Height Percentile from Standard Growth Curves							Diastolic BP (mm Hg), by Height Percentile from Standard Growth Curves						
		5%	10%	25%	50%	75%	90%	95%	5%	10%	25%	50%	75%	90%	95%
1	90th	94	95	97	98	100	102	102	50	51	52	53	54	54	55
	95th	98	99	101	102	104	106	106	55	55	56	57	58	59	59
2	90th	98	99	100	102	104	105	106	55	55	56	57	58	59	59
	95th	101	102	104	106	108	109	110	59	59	60	61	62	63	63
3	90th	100	101	103	105	107	108	109	59	59	60	61	62	63	63
	95th	104	105	107	109	111	112	113	63	63	64	65	66	67	67
4	90th	102	103	105	107	109	110	111	62	62	63	64	65	66	66
	95th	106	107	109	111	113	114	115	66	67	67	68	69	70	71
5	90th	104	105	106	108	110	112	112	65	65	66	67	68	69	69
	95th	108	109	110	112	114	115	116	69	70	70	71	72	73	74
6	90th	105	106	108	110	111	113	114	67	68	69	70	70	71	72
	95th	109	110	112	114	115	117	117	72	72	73	74	75	76	76
7	90th	106	107	109	111	113	114	115	69	70	71	72	72	73	74
	95th	110	111	113	115	116	118	119	74	74	75	76	77	78	78
8	90th	107	108	110	112	114	115	116	71	71	72	73	74	75	75
	95th	111	112	114	116	118	119	120	75	76	76	77	78	79	80
9	90th	109	110	112	113	115	117	117	72	73	73	74	75	76	77
	95th	113	114	116	117	119	121	121	76	77	78	79	80	80	81
10	90th	110	112	113	115	117	118	119	73	74	74	75	76	77	78
	95th	114	115	117	119	121	122	123	77	78	79	80	80	81	82
11	90th	112	113	115	117	119	120	121	74	74	75	76	77	78	78
	95th	116	117	119	121	123	124	125	78	79	79	80	81	82	83
12	90th	115	116	117	119	121	123	123	75	75	76	77	78	78	79
	95th	119	120	121	123	125	126	127	79	79	80	81	82	83	83
13	90th	117	118	120	122	124	125	126	75	76	76	77	78	79	80
	95th	121	122	124	126	128	129	130	79	80	81	82	83	83	84
14	90th	120	121	123	125	126	128	128	76	76	77	78	79	80	80
	95th	124	125	127	128	130	132	132	80	81	81	82	83	84	85
15	90th	123	124	125	127	129	131	131	77	77	78	79	80	81	81
	95th	127	128	129	131	133	134	135	81	82	83	83	84	85	86
16	90th	125	126	128	130	132	133	134	79	79	80	81	82	82	83
	95th	129	130	132	134	136	137	138	83	83	84	85	86	87	87
17	90th	128	129	131	133	134	136	136	81	81	82	83	84	85	85
	95th	132	133	135	136	138	140	140	85	85	86	87	88	89	89

Source: Reprinted from National High Blood Pressure Education Program Working Group on Hypertension Control in Children and Adolescents.[3]
[a]Blood pressure percentile determined by a single measurement.

Table 17. Blood Pressure Levels for the 90th and 95th Percentiles of Blood Pressure for Girls Ages 1 to 17 Years

Age	BP Percentile[a]	Systolic BP (mm Hg), by Height Percentile from Standard Growth Curves							Diastolic BP (mm Hg), by Height Percentile from Standard Growth Curves						
		5%	10%	25%	50%	75%	90%	95%	5%	10%	25%	50%	75%	90%	95%
1	90th	97	98	99	100	102	103	104	53	53	53	54	55	56	56
	95th	101	102	103	104	105	107	107	57	57	57	58	59	60	60
2	90th	99	99	100	102	103	104	105	57	57	58	58	59	60	61
	95th	102	103	104	105	107	108	109	61	61	62	62	63	64	65
3	90th	100	100	102	103	104	105	106	61	61	61	62	63	63	64
	95th	104	104	105	107	108	109	110	65	65	65	66	67	67	68
4	90th	101	102	103	104	106	107	108	63	63	64	65	65	66	67
	95th	105	106	107	108	109	111	111	67	67	68	69	69	70	71
5	90th	103	103	104	106	107	108	109	65	66	66	67	68	68	69
	95th	107	107	108	110	111	112	113	69	70	70	71	72	72	73
6	90th	104	105	106	107	109	110	111	67	67	68	69	69	70	71
	95th	108	109	110	111	112	114	114	71	71	72	73	73	74	75
7	90th	106	107	108	109	110	112	112	69	69	69	70	71	72	72
	95th	110	110	112	113	114	115	116	73	73	73	74	75	76	76
8	90th	108	109	110	111	112	113	114	70	70	71	71	72	73	74
	95th	112	112	113	115	116	117	118	74	74	75	75	76	77	78
9	90th	110	110	112	113	114	115	116	71	72	72	73	74	74	75
	95th	114	114	115	117	118	119	120	75	76	76	77	78	78	79
10	90th	112	112	114	115	116	117	118	73	73	73	74	75	76	76
	95th	116	116	117	119	120	121	122	77	77	77	78	79	80	80
11	90th	114	114	116	117	118	119	120	74	74	75	75	76	77	77
	95th	118	118	119	121	122	123	124	78	78	79	79	80	81	81
12	90th	116	116	118	119	120	121	122	75	75	76	76	77	78	78
	95th	120	120	121	123	124	125	126	79	79	80	80	81	82	82
13	90th	118	118	119	121	122	123	124	76	76	77	78	78	79	80
	95th	121	122	123	125	126	127	128	80	80	81	82	82	83	84
14	90th	119	120	121	122	124	125	126	77	77	78	79	79	80	81
	95th	123	124	125	126	128	129	130	81	81	82	83	83	84	85
15	90th	121	121	122	124	125	126	127	78	78	79	79	80	81	82
	95th	124	125	126	128	129	130	131	82	82	83	83	84	85	86
16	90th	122	122	123	125	126	127	128	79	79	79	80	81	82	82
	95th	125	126	127	128	130	131	132	83	83	83	84	85	86	86
17	90th	122	123	124	125	126	128	128	79	79	79	80	81	82	82
	95th	126	126	127	129	130	131	132	83	83	83	84	85	86	86

Source: Reprinted from National High Blood Pressure Education Program Working Group on Hypertension Control in Children and Adolescents.[3]
[a]Blood pressure percentile determined by a single measurement.

Table 18. Classification of Blood Pressure for Adults Ages 18 Years and Older [a]

Category	Blood Pressure, mm Hg		
	Systolic		Diastolic
Optimal[b]	<120	and	<80
Normal	<130	and	<85
High-normal	130–139	or	85–89
Hypertension[c]			
Stage 1	140–159	or	90–99
Stage 2	160–179	or	100–109
Stage 3	≥180	or	≥110

Source: Reprinted from Joint National Committee on Prevention, Detection, Evaluation, and Treatment of High Blood Pressure.[4]

[a] Not taking antihypertensive drugs and not acutely ill. When systolic and diastolic blood pressures fall into different categories, the higher category should be selected to classify the individual's blood pressure status.

[b] Optimal blood pressure with respect to cardiovascular risk is less than 120/80 mm Hg. However, unusually low readings should be evaluated for clinical significance.

[c] Based on the average of two or more readings taken at each of two or more visits after an initial screening.

of mild hypertension among adolescents, particularly those who are overweight and/or have a family history of high blood pressure.

Screening and Assessment

Blood Pressure

Blood pressure screening is recommended at periodic physical examinations beginning at 3 years of age (using the method described in the *Update on the Task Force Report*[3]). Screening should be repeated at subsequent health supervision visits. Correct measurement of blood pressure in children requires a cuff sized appropriately for the child's upper right arm; the right arm is preferred for consistency and for comparison with the standardized tables.[3] When an elevated systolic or diastolic blood pressure reading is first obtained, two or more measurements at a comparable level, taken consecutively over weeks or months, must be obtained before a diagnosis of hypertension is confirmed. When standardized techniques for measuring blood pressure in children and adolescents are followed, an estimated 1 percent will be found to have persistent hypertension.

Obesity

Obesity and an excess distribution of fat in the midsection of the body ("central obesity") are recognized as significant risk factors in the development of primary hypertension. Obesity in children and adolescents can be assessed through body mass index (BMI). BMI is a weight-stature index (BMI = kg/m^2) correlated with subcutaneous and total body fat in children and adolescents.

Blood Lipids

Overweight hypertensive children and adolescents generally have abnormal blood lipid levels, which increase their risk of developing cardiovascular disease as adults. It is advisable to obtain fasting blood lipid levels for all overweight children and adolescents with primary hypertension.

Dietary Factors

Dietary modifications that reduce sodium intake and encourage a healthy weight can help lower blood pressure.[5] Hypertensive children and adolescents who also have elevated blood lipid levels should be advised to modify their intake of total fat and saturated fat. Although there is some evidence that an increased intake of calcium, potassium, and magnesium and a decreased intake of caffeine will lower blood pressure, the findings are inconclusive.

The goals of dietary screening and assessment are as follows:

- Evaluate children's and adolescents' diets for nutritional adequacy, based on the dietary guidelines in the Food Guide Pyramid,[6] with particular emphasis on including milk and other dairy products, fruits, and vegetables.

- Identify regularly or frequently eaten foods that are high in sodium and/or fat, and suggest strategies for modifying the diet.

- Identify the family member(s) with the primary responsibility for purchasing food and preparing meals, to ensure their involvement in counseling sessions.

Physical Activity

Children and adolescents who are physically fit are reported to have lower blood pressure levels than those who are not physically active. Regardless of whether they are overweight, hypertensive children and adolescents can improve their blood pressure level by participating in more aerobic physical activity on a regular basis. Children and adolescents with primary hypertension typically can participate in sports and strenuous physical activity without restrictions, except for intense isometric exercise (e.g., power lifting and some weight training, which can dramatically increase blood pressure).

Health professionals should screen for physical activity by asking questions about the type, frequency, and duration of physical activity performed alone, with family members, with peers, at school, and at community recreational facilities.

The goals of physical activity screening and assessment are as follows:

- Identify age-appropriate aerobic physical activities that are acceptable, attainable, and enjoyable for the child or adolescent to pursue regularly.

- Assess the child's or adolescent's level of physical inactivity (i.e., sedentary behavior) in order to help families set appropriate limits for activities such as watching television and videotapes, playing computer games, and spending time on the telephone.

Tobacco

Nicotine exposure is associated with elevated blood pressure in adults. Thus, it is essential for hypertensive children and adolescents to avoid any form of tobacco.

Treatment

Modifying dietary and physical activity behaviors is the initial strategy used in treating primary hypertension in children and adolescents. Overweight children and adolescents with hypertension need effective weight-management strategies to improve their health. Introducing medication to lower blood pressure is considered only when the recommended changes do not significantly improve blood pressure after 6 to 12 months. If medication is prescribed, it is still important to adhere to the dietary and physical activity recommendations for primary hypertension.[3]

Sodium and Salt

The effect of dietary sodium on increased blood pressure is more pronounced in individuals who are "salt sensitive." Because there is no simple way to screen for salt sensitivity, children and adolescents with primary hypertension or those with high-normal blood pressure should be advised to follow a moderate sodium-restricted diet.[3]

Some U.S. dietary surveys have estimated sodium intake as high as 5,000 mg per day. This intake far exceeds the estimated adequate daily intake for sodium needed to support growth and development during childhood and adolescence.[7] A moderate sodium-restricted diet for children and adolescents is considered to be 1,500 to 2,500 mg per day.

To achieve this moderate intake of sodium, the following measures are advised:

- Don't add salt to food at the table.

- During cooking, omit added salt and other seasonings with sodium.

- Reduce intake of processed or packaged foods high in salt and other sodium compounds, including salted snacks (e.g., chips, pretzels, popcorn, nuts, crackers); processed cheeses; condiments (e.g., ketchup, mustard); cured meats (e.g., bacon, sausage, hot dogs, lunch meats); soups; and most commercially prepared soups and main-course foods that are frozen, boxed, or canned.

- Limit intake of foods from fast-food restaurants because some items contain one-third or more of the recommended daily sodium intake.

Physical Activity

Counseling hypertensive children and adolescents (particularly those who are sedentary and overweight) to become more active can be difficult. Helping families make regular physical activity a priority, enlisting the involvement of school physical education instructors, and using community recreational facilities all encourage children and adolescents to make physical activity an enjoyable part of their life.

References

1. National Heart, Lung, and Blood Institute, Task Force on Blood Pressure Control in Children. 1977. Report of the Task Force on Blood Pressure Control in Children. *Pediatrics* 59(52 Suppl.):I–II, 797–820.

2. National Heart, Lung, and Blood Institute, Task Force on Blood Pressure Control in Children. 1987. Report of the Second Task Force on Blood Pressure Control in Children. *Pediatrics* 79(1):1–25.

3. National Heart, Lung, and Blood Institute, National High Blood Pressure Education Program Working Group on Hypertension Control in Children and Adolescents. 1997. *Update on the Task Force Report (1987) on High Blood Pressure in Children and Adolescents: A Working Group Report from the National High Blood Pressure Education Program.* Bethesda, MD: National Heart, Lung, and Blood Institute, National High Blood Pressure Education Program Working Group on Hypertension Control in Children and Adolescents. NIH Publication No. 97-3790. [Also available in *Pediatrics,* 1996, 98(4):649–658.]

4. Joint National Committee on Prevention, Detection, Evaluation, and Treatment of High Blood Pressure. 1997. The sixth report of the Joint National Committee on Prevention, Detection, Evaluation, and Treatment of High Blood Pressure. *Archives of Internal Medicine* 158:2413–2446.

5. Kirk S, Loggie JMH. 1996. Hypertension. In Rickert VI, ed., *Adolescent Nutrition: Assessment and Management.* New York, NY: Chapman and Hall (Aspen Publishers).

6. U.S. Department of Agriculture, Human Nutrition Information Service. 1992. *The Food Guide Pyramid: A Guide to Daily Food Choices.* Hyattsville, MD: U.S. Department of Agriculture.

7. National Research Council, Commission on Life Sciences, Food and Nutrition Board, Subcommittee on the Tenth Edition of the RDAs. 1989. *Recommended Dietary Allowances* (10th ed.). Washington, DC: National Academy Press.

CHILDREN AND ADOLESCENTS WITH SPECIAL HEALTH CARE NEEDS

The Maternal and Child Health Bureau has defined children and adolescents with special health care needs as those "who have or are at increased risk for chronic physical, developmental, behavioral, or emotional conditions and who require health and related services of a type or amount beyond that required by children generally."[1]

Significance

It is estimated that approximately 18 percent of children and adolescents have a chronic condition or disability.[2] These children and adolescents are at increased risk for nutrition-related health problems because of (a) physical disorders or disabilities that may affect their ability to consume, digest, or absorb nutrients; (b) biochemical imbalances caused by long-term medications or internal metabolic disturbances; (c) psychological stress from a chronic condition or physical disorder that may affect a child's appetite and food intake; and/or (d) environmental factors, which are often controlled by parents, who may influence the child's access to and acceptance of food.

Young children with special health care needs have been found to be particularly vulnerable to nutrition problems. A screening project of infants and young children with developmental delays in the Massachusetts Early Head Start Program found that 92 percent of the infants and children had at least one nutrition risk factor, and 67 percent met more than one of the criteria for referral to nutri-

tion services.[3] Nutrition reports of children and adolescents with special health care needs estimate that up to 40 percent have nutrition risk factors that warrant a referral to a dietitian.[4,5]

Common nutrition problems in children and adolescents with special health care needs include the following:[6,7]

- Altered energy and nutrient needs (from inborn errors of metabolism)

- Delayed growth

- Feeding delays or oral-motor dysfunction

- Elimination problems

- Drug/nutrient interactions

- Appetite disturbances

- Unusual food habits (e.g., rumination)

- Early childhood caries, gum disease

Screening

As with any type of health or medical concern, early identification and treatment are important to correct, control, or prevent additional harm from a nutrition problem. Table 19 outlines basic nutrition-screening parameters and criteria for referral for children and adolescents with special health care needs.

Table 19. Nutrition-Screening Parameters and Criteria for Referral for Children and Adolescents with Special Health Care Needs

Screening Data	Criteria for Referral to a Dietitian
Anthropometric[a] Weight Height/length Weight/[height or length] Birthweight (for children < 18 months)	Weight/[height or length] ≤ 5th percentile Weight/[height or length] ≥ 95th percentile [Height or length]/age ≤ 5th percentile Inappropriate growth or weight change Birthweight ≤ 1500 g (for children < 18 months) Triceps skinfold (if atrophy of lower extremities > 85th percentile)
Biochemical Hemoglobin Hematocrit	Hemoglobin ≤ 11 g/100 dL[b] Hematocrit ≤ 34%[b]
Clinical/Medical Medical condition known to affect nutrition (e.g., vomiting, reflux), elimination problems, medications, and appetite or dental problems	A diagnosis of heart disease, cancer, diabetes mellitus, HIV/AIDS, cerebral palsy, inborn error of metabolism, cleft lip and palate, malabsorption syndrome, cystic fibrosis, renal disease, or spina bifida Recurring vomiting or reflux, chronic diarrhea or constipation, severe dental caries, early childhood caries (baby bottle tooth decay), long-term use of medications that could affect nutrition, megavitamin use, or prolonged decrease in appetite, with weight loss or growth failure
Diet/Feeding Feeding method (e.g., mouth, tube, parenteral) Therapeutic diet Feeding delays or problems Significant food aversions or allergies	Tube feeding or parenteral nutrition Therapeutic diet Inability to self-feed by age 2 years Limited diet because of food aversion or allergies
Other Parental or professional concern	Unresolved concerns regarding diet, nutrition, or growth

Source: Compiled from Screening Tool,[8] Campbell and Kelsey,[9] Cialone,[10] Nutrition Bureau,[11] and Isaacs et al.[12]

[a] Growth data should be recorded and plotted on a standard growth chart; growth charts are also available for specific conditions.
[b] Set lab levels according to your program standards.

Nutritional Adequacy

The energy and nutrient requirements of children and adolescents with special health care needs will vary according to their individual metabolic rate, activity level, and medical status. Specific energy calculations for certain metabolic conditions have been reported in the scientific literature. Some of the more common energy calculations are listed in Table 20. Once a desired energy level has been established and achieved, the child or adolescent should be routinely monitored to (1) ensure adequate nutrition for growth, development, and health; and (2) make adjustments for periods of stress and illness.

Nutrition Counseling

The goal of nutrition counseling for children and adolescents with special health care needs is to enable them to achieve optimal nutrition to support their growth, development, health, and level of functioning. Because of the complex nature of childhood neurodevelopmental and related disabilities, an interdisciplinary team approach to counseling and services is frequently needed to address multifaceted nutrition and feeding problems. In addition to dietitians, other health professionals (e.g., physicians; nurses; dentists; psychologists; social workers; occupational, physical, and speech therapists) may contribute to the child's or adolescent's nutrition plan and to the family's nutrition education.

Beyond general pediatric nutrition, the following additional topics should be discussed during nutritional assessments and counseling sessions for families of children and adolescents with special health care needs:

- *Effect of certain conditions on growth parameters.* Appropriate measuring equipment (e.g., wheelchair or chair scales, length boards) or alternative measurements (e.g., arm span or upper-arm segmental measurements, skinfold measurements) should be used to accommodate children and adolescents who cannot stand independently or cannot be evaluated with traditional assessment tools. Growth charts for specific conditions and illnesses may be useful (see the reference list of disorder-specific growth charts at the end of the chapter).

- *Physical activity and dietary intake.* Children and adolescents with special health care needs may have physical limitations that increase their risk of obesity.

- *Developmental level.* Children and adolescents with special health care needs may have developmental delays or neuromuscular problems that affect their eating skills. Some may need feeding evaluations and swallowing studies to determine the safest and most efficient method for feeding; some may require special eating equipment or modified textures; others may need tube feedings to supplement or replace oral feedings, especially if they have neurologic impairments.[20]

- *Elimination patterns.* Some children and adolescents with special health care needs have chronic elimination problems requiring medical attention. A number of factors can influence bowel function: diet, hydration, activity level, muscle tone, recent illness/health status, and use of medications. These parameters should be explored when evaluating chronic constipation or diarrhea.

Table 20. Selected Energy Calculations for Children and Adolescents with Special Health Care Needs, by Diagnosis

Medical Diagnosis	Energy Calculation
Down syndrome[13]	For children ages 5–11 years: Girls: 14.3 kcal/cm (36.3 kcal/inch) Boys: 16.1 kcal/cm (40.9 kcal/inch)
Spina bifida[14,15,16]	For children > 8 years who are minimally active: To maintain weight: 9–11 kcal/cm, or 50 percent of the RDA for a child of the same age To promote weight loss: 7 kcal/cm
Prader-Willi syndrome[17]	For all children and adolescents: To maintain growth within a growth channel: 10–11 kcal/cm To create a slow rate of weight loss and support linear growth: 8.5 kcal/cm
Cystic fibrosis[18]	For all children and adolescents: Calculate ideal weight based on height, using the pediatric growth chart. Multiply by the RDA for energy for age. Multiply by a factor of 1.3–1.5 (depending on the severity of the disease) to compensate for increased energy demands.
Pediatric HIV infection or AIDS[19]	For all children and adolescents: Minimum: Determine the weight (kg) at the 50th percentile for actual height on the weight/height grid of the pediatric growth chart. Multiply this weight (kg) by the RDA for kcal/kg based on age and sex. Maximum: Determine the weight (kg) at the 50th percentile for age on the weight/age grid of the pediatric growth chart. Multiply this weight (kg) by the RDA for kcal/kg based on age and sex.

Source: Compiled from Culley et al.,[13] Ekvall,[14] Dustrude and Prince,[15] Cloud,[16] Pipes and Powell,[17] Wooldridge,[18] and Bentler and Stanish.[19]

■ *Medications and vitamin/mineral supplements.* Many children and adolescents with special health care needs take medications that may alter their appetite, food intake, digestion, absorption, and elimination patterns. It is important to review each medication and to educate parents about drug/nutrient interactions or side effects that may affect nutrition. In addition, vitamin and mineral supplements should be reviewed for nutritional adequacy, safety, and need. Care should be taken to prevent unnecessary vitamin/mineral use and megadoses of certain nutrients.

■ *Nutrition and food assistance programs and community supports (as needed).* Children and adolescents with special health care needs may require many kinds of services and incur significant medical expenses. To effectively provide family-centered care, nutrition appointments should be available to families in their communities and should be coordinated with other medical appointments. Before prescribing dietary supplements or formulas for an infant, child, or adolescent, the health professional should make sure that the family has the necessary resources or can get assistance for obtaining these products. Resources for food assistance, special feeding equipment, and supplies for tube feedings or parenteral feedings will vary from state to state. Selected resources include the following: Title V Maternal and Child Health (MCH) program and Children with Special Health Care Needs (CSHCN) program; Special Supplemental Nutrition Program for Women, Infants and Children (WIC); medical assistance/Medicaid; Food Stamps Program; and private insurance. (See Appendix J: Nutrition Resources.)

Referral

Children and adolescents with special health care needs who have nutrition problems should be referred to a dietitian in their community, preferably to one who has experience in pediatric nutrition and disabilities. Pediatric dietitians may be located through university-affiliated programs, Title V–funded pediatric specialty clinics, pediatric units and outpatient departments of local hospitals, child development clinics, WIC clinics, dietitians in private practice, or the local pediatric and public-health nutrition practice groups of The American

Dietetic Association. Two community-based services for families of children with special health care needs are highlighted below.

Early Intervention Programs

Infants and children with special health care needs who are enrolled in early intervention programs in their communities should have access to dietitians, occupational therapists, physical therapists, and speech and language pathologists with expertise in pediatrics who can address nutrition and feeding issues. Early intervention services provide community-based interdisciplinary evaluations and therapy services for infants and children with developmental delays. These programs were established through Part C of the Individuals with Disabilities Education Act (IDEA), which lists dietitians/nutritionists as personnel qualified to provide early intervention services. Nutrition outcomes and objectives should be incorporated into the Individualized Family Service Plan (IFSP) for those children with feeding and nutrition issues.

Schools

The school system is an excellent community resource for families of children and adolescents with special health care needs. Through the National School Lunch Program and the National School Breakfast Program, children and adolescents may receive modified meals at school. Child and Adult Care Food Programs must provide meals at no extra cost for children and adolescents with special health care needs. Food substitutions and special meals to accommodate medical or special dietary needs are to be provided for children and adolescents identified by the educational system as having a disability. To receive these meal modifications,

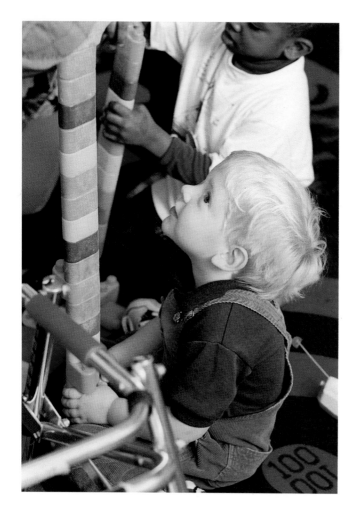

children and adolescents in special education programs must have a diet prescription on file from a health professional. The prescription must identify the disability and its effect on the child's or adolescent's diet and must state the required dietary changes and suggested meal modifications.

Children and adolescents with special health care needs who are not enrolled in a special education program must have a written order from a recognized medical authority (e.g., physician, physician assistant, nurse practitioner, or other specialist identified by the state). For children and adolescents who have chronic conditions but are not enrolled in the special education system (e.g., children with spina bifida, cerebral palsy, diabetes mellitus, or cystic fibrosis), determinations about providing modified meals are made on a case-by-case basis. To ensure that nutrition issues are addressed in the child's or adolescent's school program, nutrition goals and objectives should be incorporated in the Individualized Education Plan or 504 Accommodation Plan for children and adolescents who have significant dietary or feeding problems.[21]

References

1. McPherson M, Director, Division of Services for Children with Special Health Care Needs. August 3, 1995. Letter. Rockville, MD: Department of Health and Human Services, Health Resources and Services Administration, Maternal and Child Health Bureau.

2. Newachek P, Strickland B, Shonkoff JP, Perrin JM, McPherson M, McManus M, Lauver C, Fox M, Arrango P. 1998. An epidemiologic profile of children with special health care needs. *Pediatrics* 102(2):117–121.

3. Bayerl CT, Ries JD, Bettencourt MF, Fisher P. 1993. Nutrition issues of children in early intervention programs: Primary care team approach. *Seminars in Pediatric Gastroenterology and Nutrition* 4(1):11–15.

4. Baer MT, Farnan S, Mauer AM. 1991. Children with special health care needs. In Sharbaugh CO, with Egan MC, ed. *Call to Action: Better Nutrition for Mothers, Children, and Families—Proceedings*. Washington, DC: National Center for Education in Maternal and Child Health.

5. Hine RJ, Cloud HH, Carithers T, Hickey C, Hinton AW. 1989. Early nutrition intervention services for children with special health care needs. *Journal of The American Dietetic Association* 89(11):1636–1639.

6. American Dietetic Association. 1997. Position of The American Dietetic Association: Nutrition in comprehensive program planning for persons with developmental disabilities. *Journal of The American Dietetic Association* 97(2):189–193.

7. Dwyer JT, Freedland J. 1988. Nutrition services. In Wallace HM, Ryan Jr G, Oglesby A, eds. *Maternal and Child Health Practices* (3rd ed.). Oakland, CA: Third Party Publishing Company.

8. November 1994. Screening tool used in PHS Region IX developed under SPRANS CE Grant MCJ-009076 and MCHIP grant MCJ-065057. Los Angeles, CA: University Affiliated Program/USC, Children's Hospital. [Contacts: Baer MT, Bujold C.]

9. Campbell MK, Kelsey KE. 1994. The PEACH survey: A nutrition screening tool for use in early intervention programs. *Journal of The American Dietetic Association* 94(10):1156–1158.

10. Cialone J, Children and Youth Section, North Carolina Division of Women's and Children's Health. 1988. Nutrition screening of school age children [presentation].

11. New Mexico Health and Environmental Health, Public Health Division, Nutrition Bureau. 1987. *Criteria for Referral of Infants and Children with Handicapping Conditions for Nutrition Services.* Santa Fe, NM: New Mexico Health and Environmental Health, Public Health Division, Nutrition Bureau.

12. Isaacs JS, Cialone J, Horsley JW, Holland M, Murray P, Nardella M. 1997. *Children with Special Health Care Needs: A Community Nutrition Pocket Guide.* Birmingham, AL: University of Alabama Sparks Clinics.

13. Culley WJ, Goyal K, Jolly DH, Mertz ET. 1965. Calorie intake of children with Down syndrome. *The Journal of Pediatrics* 66(4):772–775.

14. Ekvall SW. 1993. Myelomeningocele. In Ekvall SW, ed. *Pediatric Nutrition in Chronic Diseases and Developmental Disorders: Prevention, Assessment, and Treatment.* New York, NY: Oxford University Press.

15. Dustrude A, Prince A. 1990. Provision of optimal nutrition care in myelomeningocele. *Topics in Clinical Nutrition* 5(2):34–47.

16. Cloud HH. 1993. Developmental disabilities. In Queen PA, Lang CE. *The Handbook of Pediatric Nutrition.* Gaithersburg, MD: Aspen Publishers.

17. Pipes P, Powell J. 1996. Preventing obesity in children with special health care needs. *Nutrition FOCUS for Children with Special Health Care Needs* 11(6):1–8.

18. Wooldridge NH. 1994. Nutrition management in cystic fibrosis. *Nutrition FOCUS for Children with Special Health Care Needs* 9(6):1–8.

19. Bentler M, Stanish M. 1987. Nutrition support of the pediatric patient with AIDS. *Journal of The American Dietetic Association* 87(4):488–491.

20. Lewis G, Ekvall S, Ekvall V. 1998. Neurologic handicapping conditions. In *A.S.P.E.N. Nutrition Support Practice Manual* (section 6, chapter 33, pp. 33-1–33-8). Silver Spring, MD: American Society of Parenteral and Enteral Nutrition.

21. Horsley J, Daniel PW, Allen ER. 1996. *Nutrition Management of School Age Children with Special Needs: A Resource Manual for School Personnel, Families and Health Professionals* (2nd ed.). Richmond, VA: Virginia Department of Health and Virginia Department of Education.

Suggested Reading

Acosta P, Yannicelli S. 1993. *Ross Metabolic Formula System Nutrition Support Protocol.* Columbus, OH: Ross Laboratories, Division of Abbott Laboratories USA.

The American Dietetic Association. 1995. Position of The American Dietetic Association: Nutrition services for children with special health needs. *Journal of The American Dietetic Association* 95(7):809–812.

Ekvall S, ed. 1998. *Networking in Managed Care: Providers of Nutrition Services to Individuals with Developmental/Psychiatric Disorders.* Cincinnati, OH: Cincinnati Center for Developmental Disorders.

McKinney L, Palmer C, Dwyer JT, Garcia R. 1991. Common dentally-related nutrition concerns of children with special needs. *Topics in Clinical Nutrition* 6(2):70–75.

McKinney L, Palmer C, Dwyer JT, Garcia R. 1991. Managing dentally-related nutrition concerns of children with special needs. *Topics in Clinical Nutrition* 6(2):76–85.

Stevens F, Ekvall S, eds. 1999. *Empowering Children with Cultural Diversity and Special Health Care Needs Through Early Intervention and Good Nutrition.* Cincinnati, OH: University of Cincinnati Publications.

Disorder-Specific Growth Charts

Achondroplasia

Achondroplasia Growth Charts. Skeletal Dysplasia Registry, Cedars-Sinai Medical Center, 444 South San Vicente Boulevard #1001, Los Angeles, CA 90048.

Horton WA, Rotter JI, Rimoin DL, Scott CI, Hall JG. 1978. Standard growth curves for achondroplasia. *The Journal of Pediatrics* 93(3):435–438.

Cerebral Palsy

Johnson RK, Ferrara MS. 1991. Estimating stature from knee height for persons with cerebral palsy: An evaluation of estimation equations. *Journal of The American Dietetic Association* 91(10):1283–1284.

Krick J, Murphy-Miller P, Zeger S, Wright E. 1996. Pattern of growth in children with cerebral palsy. *Journal of The American Dietetic Association* 96(7):680–685.

Spender QW, Cronk CE, Charney EB, Stallings VA. 1989. Assessment of linear growth of children with cerebral palsy: Use of alternative measures of height or length. *Developmental Medicine and Child Neurology* 31(2):206–214.

Down Syndrome

Cronk C, Crocker AC, Pueschel SM, Shea AM, Zackai E, Pickens G, Reed RB. 1988. Growth charts for children with Down syndrome: 1 month to 18 years of age. *Pediatrics* 81(1):102–110.

Fragile X Syndrome

Butler MG, Brunschwig A, Miller LK, Hagerman RJ. 1992. Standards for selected anthropometric measurements in males with fragile X syndrome. *Pediatrics* 89(6, Pt 1):1059–1062.

General

Ekvall SW, ed. 1993. *Pediatric Nutrition in Chronic Diseases and Developmental Disorders: Prevention, Assessment, and Treatment.* New York, NY: Oxford University Press.

Saul RA, Stevenson RE. 1998. *Growth References: Third Trimester through Adulthood* (2nd ed). Greenwood SC: Greenwood Genetic Center.

Muscular Dystrophy

Griffiths RD, Edwards RH. 1988. A new chart for weight control in Duchenne muscular dystrophy. *Archives of Disease in Childhood* 63(10):1256–1258.

Prader-Willi Syndrome

Butler MG, Meaney FJ. 1991. Standards for selected anthropometric measurements in Prader-Willi syndrome. *Pediatrics* 88(4):853–860.

Turner Syndrome

Lyon AF, Preece MA, Grant DB. 1985. Growth curves for girls with Turner syndrome. *Archives of Disease in Childhood* 60(10):932–935.

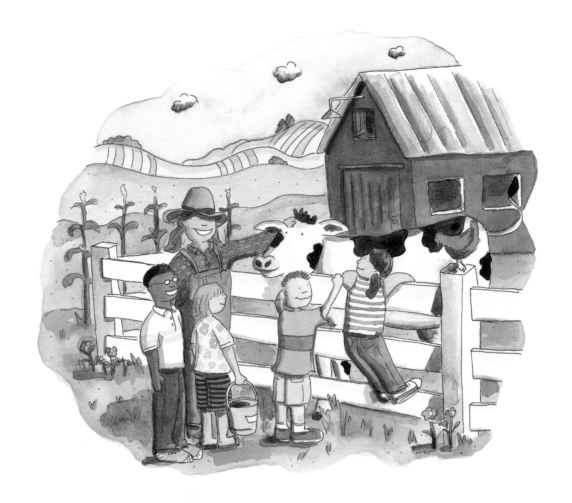

Nutrition Tools

Appendix A:
Nutrition Questionnaire for Infants

1. How would you describe feeding time with your baby? *(Circle all that apply.)*

   Always pleasant

   Usually pleasant

   Sometimes pleasant

   Never pleasant

2. How do you know when your baby is hungry or has had enough to eat?

3. What type of milk do you feed your baby? *(Circle all that apply.)*

   Breastmilk

   Iron-fortified infant formula

   Low-iron infant formula

   Goat's milk

   Evaporated milk

   Whole milk

   2 percent milk

   Low-fat milk

   Skim milk

4. What types of things can your baby do? *(Circle all that apply.)*

   Open mouth for breast or bottle

   Drink liquids

   Follow objects and sounds with eyes

   Put hand in mouth

   Sit with support

   Bring objects to mouth and bite them

   Hold bottle without support

   Drink from a cup that is held

5. Does your baby eat solid foods? If so, which ones?

6. Does your baby drink juice? If so, how much?

7. Does your baby take a bottle to bed at night or carry a bottle around during the day?

8. Do you add honey to your baby's bottle or dip your baby's pacifier in honey?

9. What is the source of the water your baby drinks? Sources include public, well, commercially bottled, and home system–processed water.

10. Do you have a working stove, oven, and refrigerator where you live?

11. Were there any days last month when your family didn't have enough food to eat or enough money to buy food?

12. What concerns or questions do you have about feeding your baby?

Interpreting the Questionnaire

This nutrition questionnaire is a tool for parents to complete before meeting with a health professional. The questionnaire provides a useful starting point for identifying areas of nutrition concern and the need for additional screening. It may be adapted with the names of foods consumed by a specific cultural group. When reviewing the responses to the questionnaire, use the interpretive notes to identify areas of concern and determine follow-up questions or actions. The notes are listed by their corresponding questions on the questionnaire.

1. Feeding is crucial for the development of a healthy relationship between parents and their infant. A parent's responsiveness to an infant's cues of hunger and satiation and the close physical contact during feeding facilitate healthy social and emotional development.

2. Signs of hunger include hand-to-mouth activity, rooting, pre-cry facial grimaces, fussing sounds, and crying. Signs of fullness are turning the head away from the nipple, showing interest in things other than eating, and closing the mouth.

3. Infants should be fed breastmilk or iron-fortified infant formula, even in infant cereal. If infants are weaned from breastmilk before 12 months, they should be fed iron-fortified infant formula rather than cow's milk. Cow's milk, goat's milk, and evaporated milk are not recommended during the first 12 months of life, and 2 percent, low-fat, and skim milk are not recommended during the first 2 years of life.

4. Developmental readiness for eating different textures of food and the acquisition of self-feeding skills are important in establishing realistic feeding goals for infants.

5. By 4 to 6 months, infants need more nutrients than can be supplied by breastmilk or infant formula alone; they should gradually be introduced to solid foods when they are developmentally ready. After the infant has accepted iron-fortified infant cereals, then fruits, vegetables, and plain, soft meats (e.g., well-cooked strained or pureed lean beef, pork, chicken, turkey) can be offered. Only one new food should be introduced at a time; parents should wait 7 or more days to see how the infant tolerates the food.

Between 6 and 12 months, infants master chewing, swallowing, and manipulation of finger foods. They begin to use cups and utensils, and while they are experimenting with new tastes and textures, their sensory and perceptual development are stimulated.

6. A reasonable amount of juice is 4 oz per day when the infant is developmentally ready (4 to 6 months or older). Juice should be served in a cup, not a bottle. It should be offered in small amounts (more than 8 to 10 oz per day is excessive) because too much juice may reduce the infant's appetite for other foods and increases the risk of loose stools and diarrhea.

7. Infants permitted to suck on a bottle of any fluid that contains carbohydrates, including juice and milk, for prolonged periods are at risk for developing early childhood caries (baby bottle tooth decay). Infants should not be put to bed at night or at naptime with a bottle or allowed unlimited access to a bottle (i.e., permitting the infant to carry a bottle around whenever he wants).

8. Honey should not be added to food, water, or formula that is fed to infants because it can be a source of spores that cause botulism poisoning in infants. Processed foods containing honey should not be given.

9. Starting at 6 months, infants receiving breastmilk or infant formula prepared with water need fluoride supplementation if the water is severely deficient in fluoride. To assess fluoride levels, ask about all sources of water used by the family, including municipal, well, commercially bottled, and home system–processed water. In addition,

find out whether any ready-to-feed infant formula used is manufactured with water that has little or no fluoride. Refer an infant who isn't getting enough fluoride to a physician or dentist for follow-up.

10–11. If inadequate cooking or food-storage facilities adversely affect a family's nutrient intake, refer the family to social services. If a family does not have adequate resources to obtain food, refer them to food assistance and nutrition programs such as WIC and the Food Stamp Program, or to a community food shelf or pantry. (See Appendix K: Federal Food Assistance and Nutrition Programs.)

12. Respond to parents' questions and concerns.

Appendix B:
Nutrition Questionnaire for Children

1. How would you describe your child's appetite?

   Good

   Fair

   Poor

2. How many days does your family eat meals together per week?

3. How would you describe mealtimes with your child?

   Always pleasant

   Usually pleasant

   Sometimes pleasant

   Never pleasant

4. How many meals does your child eat per day? How many snacks?

5. Which of these foods did your child eat or drink last week? *(Circle all that apply.)*

   Grains

   Bread

   Rolls

   Bagels

   Muffins

   Crackers

   Cereal/grits

   Noodles/pasta

   Rice

   Tortillas

   Other grains: _____

   _____

Vegetables

Corn

Peas

Potatoes

French fries

Tomatoes

Carrots

Greens (collard, spinach)

Green salad

Broccoli

Green beans

Other vegetables: _____

_____

Fruits

Apples/juice

Oranges/juice

Grapefruit/juice

Grapes/juice

Bananas

Peaches

Pears

Berries

Melon

Other fruits/juice: _____

_____

Milk and Other Dairy Products

Whole milk

2 percent milk

Low-fat milk

Skim milk

Chocolate milk

Yogurt

Cheese

Ice cream

Other milk and dairy products: _____

_____

Meat and Meat Alternatives

Beef/hamburger

Pork

Chicken

Turkey

Fish

Cold cuts/lunchmeat

Sausage/bacon

Peanut butter/nuts

Eggs

Dried beans

Tofu

Other meat and meat alternatives: _____

_____

Fats and Sweets

Cake/cupcakes

Pie

Cookies

Chips

Doughnuts

Candy

Fruit-flavored drinks

Kool-Aid

Soft drinks

Other fats and sweets: _____

_____

6. If your child is 5 years old or younger, does he or she eat any of these foods? *(Circle all that apply.)*

Hot dogs

Pretzels and chips

Raw celery or carrots

Nuts and seeds

Raisins

Whole grapes

Popcorn

Marshmallows

Round or hard candy

Peanut butter

7. How much juice does your child drink per day? How much sweetened beverage (for example, Kool-Aid, fruit punch, and soft drinks) does your child drink per day?

8. Does your child take a bottle to bed at night or carry a bottle around during the day?

9. What is the source of the water your child drinks? Sources include public, well, commercially bottled, and home system–processed water.

10. Do you have a working stove, oven, and refrigerator where you live?

11. Were there any days last month when your family didn't have enough food to eat or enough money to buy food?

12. Does your child spend more than 2 hours per day watching television and videotapes or playing computer games?

Yes   No

13. What concerns or questions do you have about feeding your child?

Interpreting the Questionnaire

This nutrition questionnaire is a tool for parents to complete before meeting with a health professional. The questionnaire provides a useful starting point for identifying areas of nutrition concern and the need for additional screening. It may be adapted with the names of foods consumed by a specific cultural group. When reviewing the responses to the questionnaire, use the interpretive notes to identify areas of concern and determine follow-up questions or actions. The notes are listed by their corresponding questions on the questionnaire.

1. Children grow more slowly from ages 1 to 5 than in infancy. Their appetites can change from day to day, depending on how fast they are growing and how active they are. As long as they are energetic and growing, they are probably getting enough of the nutrients they need. Young children often eat small portions. They should be offered small servings and be allowed to ask for more.

   Irregular eating and frequently missing meals can result in a low intake of calories (energy) and nutrients. Busy schedules and inadequate resources for obtaining food may cause a child to miss meals.

2. Encourage parents to eat meals together as a family. If children see their parents and other adults enjoying meals together and eating a variety of foods, they will want to do the same. Explain that being a role model is the best teacher.

3. During mealtimes, a relaxed atmosphere should be maintained and children should not be rushed. Well-balanced meals and snacks should be offered in a pleasant environment. When children are stubborn about eating, it is often their way of learning to be independent. Fighting over food may make them even more stubborn. Encourage parents to get rid of distractions such as television during meals.

4. Meals and snacks for children need to be planned and offered at scheduled times throughout the day and should consist of a variety of healthy foods. Children should not be pressured or rewarded to eat certain foods.

5. Children 2 to 3 years old need the variety and same number of servings as older children but may need small portions—about $2/3$ of a serving. By the time children are 4 years old, they eat portions similar to those eaten by older family members: 1 slice of bread; 1 cup of raw vegetables; 1 medium-size piece of fruit; 1 cup of milk or yogurt; 2 to 3 oz of cooked lean meat, poultry, or fish.

   Grains. Children need 6 to 11 servings per day. Grain products provide vitamins, minerals, complex carbohydrates, and dietary fiber, which are important for good health.

   Vegetables. Children need 3 to 5 servings per day. Vegetables provide vitamins, minerals, and dietary fiber. Children need to eat dark-green leafy and deep-yellow vegetables often.

   Fruits. Children need 2 to 4 servings per day. Fruits provide vitamins, minerals, and dietary fiber. Many juice beverages are not 100 percent juice. Parents need to check the ingredients to make sure that they purchase juice without added sugar such as corn syrup, and canned fruits with little or no added sugar.

   Milk and other dairy products. Children need 2 to 3 servings per day. Milk, yogurt, cheese, and other dairy products supply calcium for building and maintaining strong bones and teeth and protecting bones from osteoporosis. Children 1 to 2 years old need whole milk. Older children can drink 2 percent, low-fat, or skim milk.

   Meat and meat alternatives. Children need 2 to 3 servings per day. Meat and meat alternatives include both animal and plant sources of protein, iron, and other important nutrients. Two to 3 oz of cooked lean meat, poultry, or fish equal 1 serving from this group. One egg or $1/2$ cup of cooked dry beans counts as 1 oz of lean meat; 2 tablespoons of peanut butter count as 1 oz of meat.

Fats and sweets. This group includes butter, margarine, mayonnaise, vegetable oil, gravy, salad dressing, cake/cupcakes, pie, cookies, chips, doughnuts, and candy. There is no recommended serving because consumption of fats and sweets should be limited.

6. Young children, 2- to 3-year-olds especially, are at risk for choking on food and remain at risk until they can chew and swallow better at about age 4. Precautions to prevent choking include

   • Staying with children while they are eating.

   • Having children sit while eating because eating while walking or running can cause choking.

   • Keeping things calm at eating time because becoming overexcited while eating can cause choking.

   For children under age 2, foods that may cause choking need to be avoided (e.g., hard candy, mini-marshmallows, popcorn, pretzels, chips, spoonfuls of peanut butter, nuts, seeds, large chunks of meat, hot dogs, raw carrots, raisins and other dried fruits, whole grapes).

   For children between ages 2 and 5, foods that may cause choking can be modified to make them safer (e.g., by cutting hot dogs in quarters lengthwise and then into small pieces, cutting whole grapes in half lengthwise, chopping nuts finely, chopping raw carrots finely or into thin strips, spreading peanut butter thinly on crackers or bread).

7. Juice should be offered in small amounts because too much juice may reduce a child's appetite for meals. Parents should limit sugary drinks such as Kool-Aid, fruit punch, soft drinks, and artificially sweetened beverages. If allowed to consume sweets in unlimited amounts, children are likely to fill up on these rather than eat healthy foods.

8. Children permitted to suck on a bottle of any fluid that contains carbohydrates, including juice and milk, for prolonged periods are at risk for developing early childhood caries (baby bottle tooth decay). Children should not be put to bed at night or naptime with a bottle or allowed unlimited access to a bottle (i.e., permitting the child to carry a bottle around whenever she wants).

9. Children need fluoride supplementation if the water is severely deficient in fluoride. To assess fluoride levels, ask about all sources of water used by the family, including municipal, well, commercially bottled, and home system–processed water. Refer a child who isn't getting enough fluoride to a physician or dentist for follow-up.

10–11. If inadequate cooking or food-storage facilities adversely affect a family's nutrient intake, refer the family to social services. If a family does not have adequate resources to obtain food, refer them to food assistance and nutrition programs such as WIC and the Food Stamp Program, or to a community food shelf or pantry. (See Appendix K: Federal Food Assistance and Nutrition Programs.)

12. Children who spend too much time watching television and videotapes or playing computer games are likely to have a sedentary lifestyle, which can lead to overweight. These sedentary activities should be limited to 1 to 2 hours per day.

13. Respond to parents' questions and concerns.

Appendix C:
Nutrition Questionnaire for Adolescents

1. Which of these meals or snacks did you eat yesterday? *(Circle all that apply.)*

   Breakfast

   Morning snack

   Lunch

   Afternoon snack

   Dinner/supper

   Evening snack

2. Do you skip breakfast three or more times a week?

   Yes   No

   Do you skip lunch three or more times a week?

   Yes   No

   Do you skip dinner/supper three or more times a week?

   Yes   No

3. Do you eat dinner/supper with your family four or more times a week?

   Yes   No

4. Do you fix or buy the food for any of your family's meals?

   Yes   No

5. Do you eat or take out a meal from a fast-food restaurant two or more times a week?

   Yes   No

6. Are you on a special diet for medical reasons?

   Yes   No

7. Are you a vegetarian?   Yes   No

8. Do you have any problems with your appetite, like not feeling hungry, or feeling hungry all the time?

   Yes   No

9. Which of the following did you drink last week? *(Circle all that apply.)*

   Regular soft drinks

   Diet soft drinks

   Fruit-flavored drinks

   Kool-Aid

   Whole milk

   2 percent milk

   Low-fat milk

   Skim milk

   Chocolate milk

   Coffee/tea

   Tap/bottled water

   Orange juice

   Other juices

   Sports drinks

   Beer/wine/hard liquor

10. Which of these foods did you eat last week? *(Circle all that apply.)*

    Grains

    Bread

    Rolls

    Bagels

    Crackers

    Cereal/grits

    Popcorn

    Noodles/pasta

    Rice

    Tortillas

    Other grains: _____

    _____

Vegetables

Corn

Peas

Potatoes

French fries

Tomatoes

Carrots

Greens (collard, spinach)

Green salad

Broccoli

Green beans

Other vegetables: _____

_____

Fruits

Apples/juice

Oranges/juice

Grapefruit/juice

Grapes/juice

Bananas

Peaches

Pears

Berries

Melon

Other fruits/juice: _____

_____

Milk and Other Dairy Products

Whole milk

2 percent milk

Low-fat milk

Skim milk

Chocolate milk

Yogurt

Cheese

Ice cream

Other milk and dairy products: _____

_____

Meat and Meat Alternatives

Beef/hamburger

Pork

Chicken

Turkey

Fish

Cold cuts/lunchmeat

Sausage/bacon

Peanut butter/nuts

Eggs

Dried beans

Tofu

Other meat and meat alternatives: _____

_____

Fats and Sweets

Cake/cupcakes

Pie

Cookies

Chips

Doughnuts

Candy

Other fats and sweets: _____

_____

11. Do you have a working stove, oven, and refrigerator where you live?

Yes   No

12. Were there any days last month when your family didn't have enough food to eat or enough money to buy food?

        Yes   No

13. Are you concerned about your weight?

        Yes   No

14. Are you on a diet now to lose weight or to maintain your weight?

        Yes   No

15. In the past year, have you tried to lose weight or control your weight by vomiting, taking diet pills or laxatives, or not eating?

        Yes   No

16. On how many of the past 7 days did you participate in *moderate* physical activities (for example, walking or riding a bike) for at least 30 minutes?

17. On how many of the past 7 days did you participate in *vigorous* physical activities that made you breathe hard (for example, basketball, fast dancing, or swimming) for at least 20 minutes?

18. Do you spend more than 2 hours per day watching television and videotapes or playing computer games?

        Yes   No

19. Do you take vitamin, mineral, herbal, or other dietary supplements (for example, protein powders)?

        Yes   No

20. Do you smoke cigarettes or chew tobacco?

        Yes   No

21. Do you ever use any of the following? *(Circle all that apply.)*

Alcohol/beer/wine

Steroids (without a doctor's permission)

Street drugs (marijuana/speed/crack/heroin)

Interpreting the Questionnaire

This nutrition questionnaire is a tool for adolescents or parents to complete before meeting with a health professional. The questionnaire provides a useful starting point for identifying areas of nutrition concern and the need for additional screening. It may be adapted with the names of foods consumed by a specific cultural group. When reviewing the responses to the questionnaire, use the interpretive notes to identify areas of concern and determine follow-up questions or actions. The notes are listed by their corresponding questions on the questionnaire.

Eating Behaviors

1–2. Irregular eating and frequently missing meals can result in a low intake of calories (energy) and nutrients. Busy schedules and inadequate resources for obtaining food may cause an adolescent to miss meals. If the adolescent is overweight, reinforce the importance of eating three meals per day instead of frequent snacks.

3. Adolescents who are on their own for most meals—perhaps because of a busy schedule—may not have healthy eating behaviors. Remind adolescents and parents that family meals ensure optimal nutrition and encourage communication. Explain to parents that family meals give them the opportunity to model healthy eating behaviors.

4. Shopping for and preparing food give adolescents the opportunity to learn about healthy food choices. Make sure the adolescent is familiar with the basic rules of food safety.

5. Consumption of convenience and fast foods is common among Americans. Frequent consumption increases fat, caloric, and sodium intake and reduces the intake of certain vitamins and minerals. Suggest that adolescents reduce the consumption of these foods, and offer suggestions for making healthier food choices.

6. If the adolescent is on a special diet, ask, "What kind of diet are you on?" This will provide an opportunity to evaluate the adolescent's dietary management of conditions such as diabetes mellitus.

7. Because the term "vegetarian" is often used loosely, ask adolescents who follow a vegetarian diet which foods they eat. Further assessment is recommended.

8. Excessive or poor appetite and weight gain or loss may indicate depression or other emotional stress, which should be assessed. Because excessive appetite may also indicate binge eating or overeating, an adolescent who reports excessive appetite needs further assessment to rule out an eating disorder.

9. Soft drinks, fruit-flavored drinks, Kool-Aid, coffee, and tea contain few essential nutrients and may displace healthier beverages (e.g., milk, which provides calcium, protein, and vitamins; orange juice, which is an important source of vitamin C and folate).

Food Choices

10. *Grains.* Grains supply complex carbohydrates (which are important sources of energy), protein, and minerals; they also tend to be low in fat. Whole grains are a good source of dietary fiber. Six to 11 servings of grains per day are recommended.

    Vegetables. Vegetables provide vitamins, such as A and C, and minerals, such as calcium and iron. Most are low in fat and high in dietary fiber. Green leafy vegetables are good sources of folate. Three to 5 servings of vegetables per day are recommended.

    Fruits. Fruits are important sources of vitamins and fiber and are low in fat. Citrus fruits and juices, strawberries, and cantaloupe are good sources of vitamin C and folate. Two to 4 servings of fruits per day are recommended.

Milk and other dairy products. Milk, yogurt, and cheese are good sources of calcium and provide protein, vitamins, and minerals. Three or more servings per day of milk and other dairy products are recommended. Encourage the adolescent to consume skim or low-fat milk and other low-fat dairy products. Adequate calcium intake during adolescence is essential for peak bone-mass development. If the recommended calcium intake cannot be met by diet, a supplement may be warranted. Of the various forms of calcium, calcium carbonate contains the highest proportion (40 percent) of elemental calcium by weight.

Meat and meat alternatives. Red meat, poultry, fish, eggs, and dried beans provide protein, iron, zinc, and many other minerals and vitamins. Adequate protein intake is essential for growth and development. Two to 3 servings of meat or meat alternatives per day are recommended. Cold cuts, bacon, sausage, and fried meats are high in fat and calories; therefore, their consumption should be limited.

Fats and sweets. This group includes butter, margarine, mayonnaise, vegetable oil, gravy, salad dressing, cake/cupcakes, pie, cookies, chips, doughnuts, and candy. There is no recommended serving because consumption of fats and sweets should be limited.

Food Resources

11–12. If inadequate cooking or food-storage facilities adversely affect a family's nutrient intake, refer the family to social services. If a family does not have adequate resources to obtain food, refer the family to food assistance and nutrition programs such as the Food Stamp Program, a community food shelf or pantry, or a free or reduced-price school meal program. (See Appendix K: Federal Food Assistance and Nutrition Programs.)

Weight and Body Image

13. Some adolescents may be dissatisfied with their weight and use unhealthy means to alter it. If the adolescent expresses a concern about weight, follow up with questions such as "Do you feel you are underweight?" "Do you feel you are overweight?" "Are you doing anything to change your weight?"

14. If the adolescent is dieting, determine the frequency, duration, and methods of weight loss. Chronic food restriction and inadequate energy intake may cause poor growth, delayed sexual development, menstrual irregularities, poor concentration, irritability, sleep difficulties, and constipation. Frequent dieting may be associated with binge eating. Purging (e.g., self-induced vomiting, laxative use) may be associated with other risk behaviors (e.g., substance use, suicide attempts).

15. Self-induced vomiting and/or the use of laxatives, diuretics, or diet pills are warning signs of eating disorders. Adolescents who engage in these behaviors need further assessment.

Physical Activity

16–17. The Surgeon General's report on physical activity and health recommends 30 minutes or more of moderately intensive physical activity all or most days of the week. Longer or more vigorous physical activity will yield greater health benefits. The benefits of physical activity include weight control, cardiovascular health, and overall emotional health. Help the inactive adolescent identify enjoyable activities and incorporate them into a daily routine.

Some adolescents participate in a physical activity too frequently or intensely. Excessive physical activity may lead to fatigue, loss of appetite, or menstrual irregularities; it may also be a sign of an eating disorder.

Lifestyle

18. Adolescents who spend too much time watching television and videotapes or playing computer games are likely to have a sedentary lifestyle, which can lead to overweight. These sedentary activities should be limited to 1 to 2 hours per day.

19. If the adolescent uses vitamin, mineral, herbal, or other dietary supplements, ask about the kind, dosage, length of use, and reason for use. Encourage the adolescent to eat healthy foods instead of using supplements to obtain nutrients. If the adolescent is interested in vitamin supplements, emphasize the importance of using low-dose supplements and the need to avoid high doses (particularly of vitamins A and D), which can be toxic.

    Adolescents who participate in physical activities in which strength is a critical factor (e.g., football, weightlifting) may consume a high-protein diet or take protein supplements to increase strength and muscle mass. However, increased protein intake does not affect muscle size.

    Adolescents who use protein supplements should be asked about anabolic steroid use. Some adolescents take anabolic steroids to enhance their strength, muscle size, and endurance. Steroid use can cause side effects, including acne, deepening of the voice, and hair recession.

20. Unhealthy behaviors occur in clusters in adolescents. For example, adolescents who smoke are more likely to have unhealthy eating behaviors and low levels of physical activity. Adolescents who smoke cigarettes to lose weight need counseling on both smoking and healthy weight management. Cigarette smoking also increases the need for vitamin C.

21. If the adolescent admits to using alcohol or street drugs, screen for substance use and refer for counseling and treatment.

    Some adolescents take anabolic steroids to enhance their strength, muscle size, and endurance. Steroid use can cause side effects, including acne, deepening of the voice, and hair recession. Emphasize the dangers of steroid use to adolescents who participate in strenuous physical activity to build muscle or who engage in sports in which strength is a critical factor (e.g., football, weightlifting).

Appendix D: Key Indicators of Nutrition Risk for Children and Adolescents

Indicators of Nutrition Risk	Relevance	Criteria for Further Screening and Assessment
Food Choices		
Consumes fewer than 2 servings of fruit or fruit juice per day. Consumes fewer than 3 servings of vegetables per day.	Fruits and vegetables provide dietary fiber, vitamins (such as A and C), and minerals. Low intake of fruits and vegetables is associated with an increased risk of many types of cancer. In females of childbearing age, low intake of folic acid is associated with increased risk of giving birth to an infant with neural tube defects.	Assess the child/adolescent who is consuming less than 1 serving of fruit or fruit juice per day. Assess the child/adolescent who is consuming fewer than 2 servings of vegetables per day.
Consumes fewer than 6 servings of bread, cereal, rice, pasta, or other grains per day.	Grain products provide complex carbohydrates, dietary fiber, vitamins, and minerals. Low intake of dietary fiber is associated with constipation and increased risk of colon cancer.	Assess the child/adolescent who is consuming fewer than 3 servings of bread, cereal, pasta, rice, or other grains per day. Assess the child/adolescent who has recent history of constipation.
For children younger than 9 years, consumes fewer than 2 servings of dairy products per day. For children 9 years and older and adolescents, consumes fewer than 3 servings of dairy products per day.	Dairy products are a good source of protein, vitamins, and calcium and other minerals. Low intake of dairy products may reduce peak bone mass and increase the risk of osteoporosis.	Assess the child (younger than 9 years) who is consuming less than 1 serving of dairy products per day. Assess the child (9 years and older) or adolescent who is consuming fewer than 2 servings of dairy products per day. Assess the child/adolescent who has a milk allergy or is lactose intolerant. Assess the child/adolescent who is consuming more than 2 soft drinks per day.

Indicators of Nutrition Risk	Relevance	Criteria for Further Screening and Assessment
Food Choices (cont.)		
Consumes fewer than 2 servings of meat or meat alternatives (e.g., beans, eggs, nuts, seeds) per day.	Protein-rich foods (e.g., meats, beans, dairy products) are good sources of B vitamins, iron, and zinc. Low intake of protein-rich foods may impair growth and increase the risk of iron-deficiency anemia and of delayed growth and sexual maturation. Low intake of meat or meat alternatives may indicate inadequate availability of these foods at home. Special attention should be paid to children and adolescents who follow a vegetarian diet.	Assess the child/adolescent who is consuming less than 1 serving of meat or meat alternatives per day.
For children 5 years and older, has excessive intake of dietary fat.	Excessive intake of dietary fat contributes to the risk of cardio-vascular disease and obesity and is associated with some cancers.	Assess the child/adolescent who has a family history of premature cardiovascular disease. Assess the child/adolescent who has a body mass index (BMI) greater than or equal to the 85th percentile.
Eating Behaviors		
Exhibits poor appetite.	A poor appetite may be developmentally appropriate for young children, but in older children it may indicate depression or other emotional stress or chronic disease.	Assess the child/adolescent if BMI is less than the 15th percentile or if weight loss has occurred. Assess if irregular menses or amenorrhea has occurred for 3 months or more. Assess for organic and psychiatric disease.
Consumes food from fast-food restaurants 3 or more times per week.	Excessive consumption of convenience foods and foods from fast-food restaurants is associated with high fat, calorie, and sodium intake, as well as low intake of certain vitamins and minerals.	Assess the child/adolescent who is overweight/obese or who has diabetes mellitus, hyperlipidemia, or other conditions requiring reduction in dietary fat.

Indicators of Nutrition Risk	Relevance	Criteria for Further Screening and Assessment
Eating Behaviors (cont.)		
Skips breakfast, lunch, or dinner/supper 3 or more times per week.	Meal skipping is associated with a low intake of energy and essential nutrients and, if it is a regular practice, could compromise growth and sexual development. Repeatedly skipping meals decreases the nutritional adequacy of the diet.	Assess the child/adolescent to ensure that meal skipping is not due to inadequate food resources or unhealthy weight-loss practices.
Has food jags—eats one particular food only.	Food jags, which limit the variety of food consumed, decrease the nutritional adequacy of the diet.	Assess the child's/adolescent's dietary intake over several days.
Food Resources		
Has inadequate financial resources to buy food, insufficient access to food, or lack of access to cooking facilities.	Poverty can result in hunger and compromised food quality and nutrition status. Inadequate dietary intake interferes with learning.	Assess the child/adolescent who is from a family with low income, is homeless, or is a runaway. (See Appendix K: Federal Food Assistance and Nutrition Programs.)
Weight and Body Image		
Practices unhealthy behaviors (e.g., chronic dieting, vomiting, and using laxatives, diuretics, or diet pills to lose weight).	Chronic dieting is associated with many health concerns (e.g., fatigue, impaired growth and sexual maturation, irritability, poor concentration, impulse to binge) and can lead to eating disorders. Frequent dieting in combination with purging is associated with health-compromising behaviors (e.g., substance use, suicidal behaviors). Purging is associated with serious medical complications.	Assess the child/adolescent for eating disorders. Assess for organic and psychiatric disease.
Is excessively concerned about body size or shape.	Eating disorders are associated with significant health and psychosocial morbidity. Eighty-five percent of all cases of eating disorders begin during adolescence. The earlier adolescents are treated, the better their long-term prognosis.	Assess the child/adolescent for distorted body image and dysfunctional eating behaviors, especially if child/adolescent wants to lose weight but BMI is less than the 85th percentile.

Indicators of Nutrition Risk	Relevance	Criteria for Further Screening and Assessment
Weight and Body Image (cont.)		
Exhibits significant weight change in past 6 months.	Significant weight change during the past 6 months may indicate stress, depression, organic disease, or an eating disorder.	Assess the child/adolescent to determine the cause of weight loss or weight gain (e.g., limited or too much access to food, poor appetite, meal skipping, eating disorder).
Growth		
Has BMI less than the 5th percentile.	Thinness may indicate an eating disorder or poor nutrition.	Assess the child/adolescent for eating disorders. Assess for organic or psychiatric disease. Assess for inadequate food resources.
Has BMI greater than the 95th percentile.	Obesity is associated with elevated cholesterol levels and elevated blood pressure. Obesity is an independent risk factor for cardiovascular disease and type 2 diabetes mellitus in adults. Overweight children and adolescents are more likely to be overweight adults and are at increased risk for health problems as adults.	Assess the child/adolescent who is overweight or at risk for becoming overweight (e.g., on the basis of present weight, weight gain patterns, family weight history).
Physical Activity		
Is physically inactive: engages in physical activity fewer than 5 days per week.	Lack of physical activity is associated with overweight, fatigue, and poor muscle tone in the short term, and a greater risk of cardiovascular disease in the long term. Regular physical activity reduces the risk of cardiovascular disease, hypertension, colon cancer, and type 2 diabetes mellitus. Weight-bearing physical activity is essential for normal skeletal development during childhood. Regular physical activity is necessary for maintaining normal muscle strength, joint structure, and joint function; contributes to psychological health and well-being; and facilitates weight reduction and weight maintenance throughout life.	Assess how much time the child/adolescent spends watching television/videotapes and playing computer games. Assess the child's/adolescent's definition of physical activity.

Indicators of Nutrition Risk	Relevance	Criteria for Further Screening and Assessment
Physical Activity (cont.)		
Engages in excessive physical activity.	Intense physical activity nearly every day, sometimes more than once a day, can be unhealthy and associated with menstrual irregularity, excessive weight loss, and malnutrition.	Assess the child/adolescent for eating disorders.
Medical Conditions		
Has chronic diseases or conditions.	Medical conditions (e.g., diabetes mellitus, spina bifida, renal disease, hypertension, pregnancy, HIV infection/AIDS) have significant nutritional implications.	Assess child's/adolescent's compliance with therapeutic dietary recommendations. Refer to dietitian if appropriate.
Has hyperlipidemia.	Hyperlipidemia is a major cause of atherosclerosis and cardiovascular disease in adults.	Refer child/adolescent to a dietitian for cardiovascular nutrition assessment.
Has iron-deficiency anemia.	Iron deficiency causes developmental delays and behavioral disturbances. Another consequence is increased lead absorption. Childhood lead poisoning causes neurological and developmental deficits.	Screen children whose families have low incomes, are migrant, or are recently arrived refugees. Screen male children/adolescents who have low iron intake, a history of iron-deficiency anemia, limited access to food because of poverty or neglect, or special health care needs. Screen nonpregnant adolescents every 5 to 10 years or annually if they have a history of iron-deficiency anemia, low iron intake, or extensive menstrual or other blood loss.

Indicators of Nutrition Risk	Relevance	Criteria for Further Screening and Assessment
Medical Conditions (cont.)		
Has dental caries.	Food affects the health of the mouth as well as overall health. Calcium and vitamin D are vital for strong bones and teeth, and vitamin C is necessary for healthy gums. Eating habits have a direct impact on oral health. Frequent consumption of carbohydrate-rich foods (e.g., lollipops, soda) that stay in the mouth longer may cause dental caries. Fluoride in water used for drinking and cooking as well as in toothpaste reduces the prevalence of dental caries.	Assess the child's/adolescent's consumption of snacks and beverages that contain sugar, and assess snacking patterns. Assess the child's/adolescent's access to fluoride (e.g., fluoridated water, fluoride tablets).
Is pregnant.	Pregnancy increases the need for most nutrients.	Refer the adolescent to a dietitian for further assessment, education, and counseling as appropriate.
Is taking prescription medication.	Many medications interact with nutrients and can compromise nutrition status.	Assess potential interactions of prescription drugs (e.g., asthma medications, antibiotics) with nutrients.
Lifestyle		
Engages in heavy alcohol, tobacco, and other drug use.	Alcohol, tobacco, and other drug use can adversely affect nutrient intake and nutrition status.	Assess the child/adolescent further for alcohol, tobacco, and other drug use.
Uses dietary supplements.	Dietary supplements (e.g., vitamin and mineral preparations) can be healthy additions to a diet, especially for pregnant and lactating women and for people with a history of iron-deficiency anemia; however, frequent use or high doses can have serious side effects. Adolescents who use supplements to "bulk up" may be tempted to experiment with anabolic steroids.	Assess the child/adolescent for the type of supplements used and dosages. Assess the adolescent for use of anabolic steroids and megadoses of other supplements.

Appendix E: Screening for Elevated Blood Lead Levels

In 1997, the Centers for Disease Control and Prevention (CDC) updated its lead screening guidelines and published revised guidance to help state and local public health authorities determine which children are at risk for elevated blood lead levels and are most likely to benefit from lead screening.[1] The American Academy of Pediatrics (AAP) supports these revised guidelines. The following information has been compiled from CDC and AAP guidelines.[1,2] Federal Medicaid policy requires that all eligible children be screened for lead poisoning as described below under Universal Screening, because they are at high risk for lead poisoning.

Screening Recommendations

To prevent lead poisoning, lead screening should begin at 9 to 12 months of age and be considered again at approximately 24 months of age. Health professionals should follow the local or state health department recommendations for universal or targeted screening.[2]

Universal Screening

Universal screening will be recommended in communities in which the risk of lead exposure is widespread. A universal screening recommendation may read as follows:[1(p85)]

Using a blood lead test, screen all children at ages 1 and 2, and all children 36–72 months of age who have not been previously screened.

Targeted Screening

Targeted screening will be recommended in communities in which the risk of lead exposure is not widespread or is confined to specific geographic areas or to certain subpopulations. Health professionals should determine whether each child is at risk and screen when necessary. A sample targeted screening recommendation follows:[1(p85)]

Using a blood lead test, screen children at ages 1 and 2, and all children 36–72 months of age who have not been previously screened, if they meet one of the following health department criteria:

- Child resides in a geographic area (e.g., a specified zip code) in which ≥ 27 percent of housing was built before 1950

- Child receives services from public assistance programs such as Medicaid or WIC

- Child's parent or guardian answers "yes" or "don't know" to any of the three questions in the basic personal-risk questionnaire

---

A Basic Personal-Risk Questionnaire for Lead Exposure in Children

1. Does your child live in or regularly visit a house or child-care facility that was built before 1950?

2. Does your child live in or regularly visit a house or child-care facility built before 1978 that is being or has recently been renovated or remodeled (within the last 6 months)?

3. Does your child have a sibling or playmate who has or did have lead poisoning?

Source: Reproduced with permission from AAP.[2] Copyright © 1998 American Academy of Pediatrics. See also CDC.[1(p62)]

History of Possible Lead Exposure

Health professionals should periodically assess infants and children between 6 months and 6 years of age for a history of possible lead exposure, using the basic personal-risk questionnaire here and any additional community-specific questions recommended by the state or local health department. Blood lead testing should also be considered in abused or neglected children and in children who have conditions associated with increased lead exposure.[2]

APPENDIX E

Table E1. Risk Factors and Prevention Strategies for Lead Exposure in Children

Risk Factor	Prevention Strategy
Environmental	
Lead-based paint	Identify and abate
Dust	Use a wet mop to clean; wash hands frequently
Soil	Restrict play in area; plant ground cover; wash hands frequently
Drinking water	Flush water for 2 minutes before using in morning; use cold water for cooking, drinking
Folk remedies	Avoid use
Old ceramic or pewter cookware, old urns/kettles	Avoid use
Some imported cosmetics, toys, crayons	Avoid use
Parental occupations	Remove work clothing at work
Hobbies	Ensure the proper use, storage, and ventilation of materials
Home renovation	Ensure the proper containment of building hazards and proper ventilation
Buying or renting a new home	Inquire about lead hazards
Host	
Hand-to-mouth activity (or pica)	Wash hands frequently
Inadequate nutrition	Ensure that diet is high in iron and calcium and low in fat; eat frequent small meals
Developmental disabilities	Screen frequently for lead exposure

Source: Adapted with permission from AAP.[2] Copyright © 1998 American Academy of Pediatrics.

Anticipatory Guidance

Health professionals should provide anticipatory guidance on lead exposure to parents of all infants and young children, including information on risk factors and specific prevention strategies (Table E1).[2] CDC recommends providing anticipatory guidance at prenatal visits, when the infant is 3 to 6 months of age, and again at 12 months of age; parental guidance at these times might prevent some lead exposure and the resulting increase in blood lead levels that often occurs during a child's second year of life. When children are 1 to 2 years old, parental guidance should be provided at health supervision visits and when the personal-risk questionnaire is administered.[1(p83)]

References

1. Centers for Disease Control and Prevention. 1997. *Screening Young Children for Lead Poisoning: Guidance for State and Local Public Health Officials*. Atlanta, GA: Centers for Disease Control and Prevention. Also in Centers for Disease Control and Prevention [Web site]. Cited May 14, 1999; available at http://www.cdc.gov/nceh/programs/lead/guide/1997/guide97.htm.

2. American Academy of Pediatrics. 1998. Screening for elevated blood lead levels [policy statement no. RE9815]. *Pediatrics* 101(6):1072–1078. Also in American Academy of Pediatrics [Web site]. Cited May 14, 1999; available at http://www.aap.org/policy/re9815.html.

Appendix F: Stages of Change—
A Model for Nutrition Counseling

Stage	Description	Goals	Strategies
Precontemplation	Is unaware of problem and hasn't thought about change. Has no intention of taking action within the next 6 months.	Increase awareness of need for change. Personalize information on risks and benefits.	Create supportive climate for change. Discuss personal aspects and health consequences of poor eating or sedentary behavior. Assess knowledge, attitudes, and beliefs. Build on existing knowledge.
Contemplation	Intends to take action within the next 6 months.	Increase motivation and confidence to perform the new behavior.	Identify problematic behaviors. Prioritize behaviors to change. Discuss motivation. Identify barriers to change and possible solutions. Suggest small, achievable steps to make a change.
Preparation	Intends to take action within the next 30 days and has taken some behavioral steps in this direction.	Initiate change.	Assist in developing a concrete action plan. Encourage initial small steps to change. Discuss earlier attempts to change and ways to succeed. Elicit support from family and friends.
Action	Has changed overt behavior for less than 6 months.	Commit to change.	Reinforce decision. Reinforce self-confidence. Assist with self-monitoring, feedback, problem solving, social support, and reinforcement. Discuss relapse and coping strategies.
Maintenance	Has changed overt behavior for more than 6 months.	Reinforce commitment and continue changes/new behaviors.	Plan follow-up to support changes. Help prevent relapse. Assist in coping, reminding, finding alternatives, and avoiding slips/relapses.

Source: Adapted from Glanz K, Rimer B. 1995. *Theory at a Glance: A Guide for Health Promotion Practice.* Bethesda, MD: National Institutes of Health, National Cancer Institute. Also adapted, with permission, from Sandoval WM, Heller KE, Wiese WH, Childs DA. 1994. Stages of change: A model for nutrition counseling. *Topics in Clinical Nutrition* 9:64–69. Copyright © 1994 Aspen Publishers, Inc.

Appendix G: Strategies for Health Professionals to Promote Healthy Eating Behaviors

Strategies	Applications/Questions
Communication Factors	
Promote positive, nonjudgmental strategies to help the child/adolescent adopt healthy eating behaviors.	Reinforce positive aspects of the child's/adolescent's eating behaviors.
Encourage the child's/adolescent's active participation in changing eating behaviors.	Help the child/adolescent identify barriers that make it difficult to change eating behaviors, and develop a plan of action for adopting new behaviors.
Provide concrete learning situations.	Use charts, food models, and videotapes to reinforce verbal information and instructions.
Focus on the short-term benefits of healthy eating behaviors.	Emphasize that healthy eating behaviors will make the child/adolescent feel good and energized.
Understand and respect the child's/adolescent's cultural eating behaviors.	Help the child/adolescent integrate cultural eating behaviors with dietary recommendations.
Use simple terminology.	Avoid using the term "diet" with the child/adolescent because it tends to be associated with weight loss and may be confusing.
Environmental Factors	
Provide an office or clinic oriented to children/adolescents.	Use posters and materials written for children/adolescents.
Communicate developmentally appropriate health messages.	Use posters and materials that highlight the importance of healthy eating behaviors.
Encourage health professionals and staff to become role models for healthy eating behaviors.	Have health professionals and staff model healthy eating behaviors (e.g., by keeping a bowl of fruit at the front desk).

Strategies	Applications/Questions
Readiness to Change	
Identify the child's/adolescent's stage of behavior change and readiness to change based on the Stages of Change: A Model for Nutrition Counseling (Appendix F).	"Are you interested in changing your eating behaviors?" "Are you thinking about changing your eating behaviors?" "Are you ready to change your eating behaviors?" "Are you in the process of changing your eating behaviors?" "Are you trying to maintain changes in your eating behaviors?"
Facilitate behavior change with counseling strategies tailored to the child/adolescent based on the Stages of Change model (Appendix F).	Provide a supportive environment, basic information, and assessment. Prioritize behaviors to be changed, set goals, and identify barriers to change. Develop a plan that incorporates incremental steps for making changes, support, and reinforcement.
Action Plans	
Provide counseling for the child/adolescent who is in the early stages of behavior change or who is unwilling to change.	Increase the child's/adolescent's awareness and knowledge of eating behaviors. Encourage the child/adolescent to make behavior changes if necessary.
Provide task-oriented counseling for the child/adolescent who is ready to change eating behaviors.	Encourage a few small, concrete changes first, and build on those. Support and follow up with the child/adolescent who has changed behavior.
Identify and prioritize behavior changes to be made.	Suggest changes that will have a measurable impact on the child's/adolescent's most serious nutrition issues.
Set realistic, achievable goals that are supported by the child's/adolescent's family and peers.	"What behavior will you change?" "What goal is realistic right now?" "How and when will you change the behavior and who will help you?"
Identify and address barriers to behavior change; help reduce barriers when possible.	"What will make it hard for you to make this change?" "Money, friends, or family?" "How can you get around this?"

Strategies	Applications/Questions
Action Plans (cont.)	
Make sure that the behavior changes are compatible with the child's/adolescent's lifestyle.	Don't force the child/adolescent to conform to rigid eating behaviors. Keep in mind current behaviors and realistic goals.
Establish incremental steps to help the child/adolescent change eating behaviors.	For example, have the child/adolescent reduce fat consumption by changing the type of milk consumed, from 2 percent, to low-fat, to skim milk.
Encourage the child/adolescent to commit to behavior changes with incentives or contracts.	Offer tangible non-food rewards to help the child/adolescent focus on changing eating behaviors.
Give the child/adolescent responsibility for changing and monitoring eating behaviors.	Stress the importance of planning how the child/adolescent will make and track changes in eating behavior. Make recordkeeping simple, and review the plan with the child/adolescent.
Make sure that the child/adolescent has family and peer support.	Show the child/adolescent how to encourage parents and peers to help. Meet with parents to clarify goals and action plans; determine how they can help.
Offer feedback and reinforce successes.	Regularly show interest to encourage continued behavior change.
General Strategies	
Ask the child/adolescent about changes in eating behaviors at every visit.	"How are you doing in changing your eating behaviors?"
Emphasize to the child/adolescent the consumption of foods rather than nutrients.	For example, say, "Consume more milk, cheese, and yogurt" rather than "Increase your calcium intake."
Build on positive aspects of the child's/adolescent's eating behaviors.	"It's great that you're eating breakfast. Would you be willing to try cereal, fruit, and toast instead of bacon and doughnuts 4 days out of the week?"
Focus on "how to" instead of "why" information.	Share behaviorally oriented information (e.g., what, how much, and when to eat and how to prepare food) rather than focusing on why the information is important.
Provide counseling that integrates realistic behavior change into the child's/adolescent's lifestyle.	"I understand that your friends eat lunch at fast-food restaurants. Would it help you to learn how to make healthier food choices at these restaurants?"

Strategies	Applications/Questions
General Strategies (cont.)	
Discuss how to make healthy food choices in a variety of settings.	Talk about how to choose foods in various settings such as fast-food and other restaurants, convenience stores, vending machines, and friends' homes.
Provide the child/adolescent with learning experiences and skills practice.	Practice problem solving and role-playing (e.g., having the child/adolescent ask the food server to hold the mayonnaise).
Introduce the concept of achieving balance and enjoying all foods in moderation.	"Your food record indicates that after having pepperoni pizza for lunch yesterday, you ate a lighter dinner. That's a good way to balance your food intake throughout the day."
Make recordkeeping easy, and tell the child/adolescent that you do not expect spelling, handwriting, and eating behaviors to be perfect.	"Be as accurate and honest as you can as you record your food intake. This record is a tool to help you reflect on your eating behaviors."
Make sure that the child/adolescent hears what you are saying.	"What eating behaviors are you planning to work on before your next appointment?"
Make sure that you and the child/adolescent define terms the same way to avoid confusion.	Discuss the definition of words that may cause confusion, such as "fat," "calories," "meal," and "snack."
When assessing food intake, keep in mind that a child's/adolescent's portion size may not be the same as a standard serving size.	Use food models or household cups and bowls to clarify serving sizes.

Appendix H: Tips for Promoting Food Safety

Keep Everything Clean

- Wash your hands before preparing or eating food and after anything that interrupts either of those activities.

- Wash fresh fruits and vegetables carefully before cooking or eating them raw.

- Wash dishes in a dishwasher, or wash them thoroughly in hot soapy water. Use clean dishcloths to wash dishes. Don't use sponges—they often spread germs. Rinse and sanitize dishes and let them air-dry.

- If you use a cutting board, wash it thoroughly with hot soapy water between uses for different foods, especially after using it to cut raw meat. Use cutting boards made only of nonporous materials.

Prepare Foods Properly

- Always cook foods thoroughly. Be especially careful about foods containing meat, poultry, fish, or eggs. Cook hamburger until it is brown or gray on the inside. Cook chicken until the juices are clear when a knife or fork is stuck into it. Cook fish until it is opaque and flakes easily with a fork. Cook eggs until they are firm.

- Thaw frozen foods in the refrigerator or under cold running water—*never* on the counter or in a bowl of standing water.

- Serve hot foods hot and cold foods cold. Make sure that hot foods stay above 140°F and cold foods stay below 40°F.

Store Food Safely

- If you have stored cooked foods in the refrigerator, serve them within 24 hours.

- Store raw foods below cooked or ready-to-eat foods in the refrigerator.

- Store dry ingredients (e.g., rice, sugar) in nonporous containers with tight-fitting lids to keep out insects and rodents.

- Cover and refrigerate or freeze extra cooked food right away. *Never* leave it on a counter to cool.

- Leftovers that are refrigerated or frozen should be reheated and reused only one time. If they are not all eaten the second time, throw them out.

- When you are reheating food, bring liquids such as gravy, soup, or sauce to a boil. Heat other leftovers to 165°F.

- Store cleaning products and medications away from food and out of the reach of children.

Source: Graves DE, Suitor CW, Holt KA, eds. 1997. *Making Food Healthy and Safe for Children: How to Meet the National Health and Safety Performance Standards—Guidelines for Out-of-Home Child Care Programs.* Arlington, VA: National Center for Education in Maternal and Child Health.

Appendix I: Tips for Fostering a Positive Body Image Among Children and Adolescents

Child or Adolescent	Parents	Health Professional
Look in the mirror and focus on your positive features, not the negative ones. Say something nice to your friends about how they look. Think about your positive traits that are not related to appearance. Read magazines with a critical eye, and find out what photographers and computer graphic designers do to make models look the way they do. If you are overweight and want to lose weight, be realistic in your expectations and aim for gradual change. Realize that everyone has a unique size and shape. If you have questions about your size or weight, ask a health professional.	Demonstrate healthy eating behaviors, and avoid extreme eating behaviors. Focus on non–appearance-related traits when discussing yourself and others. Praise your child or adolescent for academic and other successes. Analyze media messages with your child or adolescent. Demonstrate that you love your child or adolescent regardless of what he weighs. If your child or adolescent is overweight, don't criticize her appearance—offer support instead. Share with a health professional any concerns you have about your child's or adolescent's eating behaviors or body image.	Discuss changes that occur during adolescence. Assess weight concerns and body image. If a child or adolescent has a distorted body image, explore causes and discuss potential consequences. Discuss how the media negatively affects a child's or adolescent's body image. Discuss the normal variation in body sizes and shapes among children and adolescents. Educate parents, physical education instructors, and coaches about realistic and healthy body weight. Emphasize the positive characteristics (appearance- and non–appearance-related) of children and adolescents you see. Take extra time with an overweight child or adolescent to discuss psychosocial concerns and weight control options. Refer children, adolescents, and parents with weight control issues to a dietitian.

Appendix J: Nutrition Resources

General and federal nutrition resources are listed first, followed by resources for specific nutrition issues and concerns.

General Nutrition Information

American Academy of Family Physicians
11400 Tomahawk Creek Parkway
Leawood, KS 66211-2672
Tel: (913) 906-6000
Fax: (913) 906-6075
Web site: http://aafp.org

American Academy of Pediatrics
141 Northwest Point Boulevard
Elk Grove Village, IL 60007-1098
Tel: (847) 228-5005
Fax: (847) 228-5097
Web site: http://www.aap.org

American Cancer Society
1599 Clifton Road, N.E.
Atlanta, GA 30329-4251
Tel: (404) 320-3333, (800) 227-2345
Fax: (404) 329-7530
Web site: http://www.cancer.org

American College of Obstetricians and Gynecologists
409 12th Street, S.W.
Washington, DC 20024-2188
Tel: (202) 638-5577
Fax: (202) 484-5107
Web site: http://www.acog.org

The American Dietetic Association
216 West Jackson Boulevard, Suite 800
Chicago, IL 60606-6995
Tel: (312) 899-0040, R.D. Referral (312) 366-1655
Fax: (312) 899-4757
Web site: http://www.eatright.org

American Medical Association
515 North State Street
Chicago, IL 60610
Tel: (312) 464-5000
Fax: (312) 464-4184
Web site: http://www.ama-assn.org

American Nurses Association
600 Maryland Avenue, S.W., Suite 100 West
Washington, DC 20024-2571
Tel: (202) 651-7000
Fax: (202) 651-7001
Web site: http://nursingworld.org

American Psychological Association
750 First Street, N.E.
Washington, DC 20002-4242
Tel: (202) 336-5500
Fax: (202) 336-6069
Web site: http://www.apa.org

American Public Health Association
800 I Street, N.W.
Washington, DC 20001-3710
Tel: (202) 777-APHA
Fax: (202) 777-2534
Web site: http://www.apha.org

American School Food Services Association
700 South Washington Street, Suite 300
Alexandria, VA 22314
Tel: (703) 739-3900, (800) 877-8822
Fax: (703) 739-3915
Web site: http://www.asfsa.org

American School Health Association
Food and Nutrition Council
7263 State Route 43, P.O. Box 708
Kent, OH 44240-0708
Tel: (330) 678-1601
Fax: (330) 678-4526
Web site: http://www.ashaweb.org

Association of State and Territorial
Public Health Nutrition Directors
P.O. Box 7018
York, PA 17404-0018
Tel and fax: (717) 764-7938
Web site: http://www.astho.org

Center for Science in the Public Interest
1875 Connecticut Avenue, N.W., Suite 300
Washington, DC 20009-5728
Tel: (202) 332-9110
Fax: (202) 265-4954
Web site: http://www.cspinet.org

Consumer Information Center
1800 F Street, N.W., Room G-142, (XC)
Washington, DC 20405
Tel: (202) 501-1794
Fax: (202) 501-4281
Web site: http://www.pueblo.gsa.gov

Food and Nutrition Board
Institute of Medicine
2101 Constitution Avenue, N.W.
Washington, DC 20418
Tel: (202) 334-1732
Fax: (202) 334-2316
Web site: http://www4.nationalacademies.org/
iom/iomhome.nsf/pages/food+and+nutrition+board

Food Research and Action Center
1875 Connecticut Avenue, N.W., Suite 540
Washington, DC 20009
Tel: (202) 986-2200
Fax: (202) 986-2525
Web site: http://www.afj.org/mem/frac.html

International Food Information Council
1100 Connecticut Avenue, N.W., Suite 430
Washington, DC 20036
Tel: (202) 296-6540
Fax: (202) 296-6547
Web site: http://ificinfo.health.org

International Life Sciences Institute
1126 16th Street, N.W., Suite 300
Washington, DC 20036
Tel: (202) 659-0074
Fax: (202) 659-3859
Web site: http://www.ilsi.org

National Association of Pediatric Nurse Associates
and Practitioners
1101 Kings Highway, North, Suite 206
Cherry Hill, NJ 08034-1912
Tel: (856) 667-1773, (877) 662-7627
Fax: (856) 667-7187
Web site: http://www.napnap.org

National Association of Social Workers
750 First Street, N.E., Suite 700
Washington, DC 20002
Tel: (202) 408-8600
Fax: (202) 336-8311
Web site: http://www.socialworkers.org

National Association of WIC Directors
2001 S Street, N.W., Suite 580
Washington, DC 20009-3355
Tel: (202) 232-5492
Fax: (202) 387-5281
Web site: http://www.wicdirectors.org

National Center for Education in Maternal
  and Child Health
2000 15th Street, North, Suite 701
Arlington, VA 22201-2617
Tel: (703) 524-7802
Fax: (703) 524-9335
Web site: http://www.ncemch.org

National Center for Nutrition and Dietetics
The American Dietetic Association
216 West Jackson Boulevard
Chicago, IL 60606-6995
Tel: (312) 899-4739
Fax: (312) 899-1739
Web site: http://www.eatright.org/ncnd.html

National Center for Youth Law
405 14th Street, 15th Floor
Oakland, CA 94612
Tel: (510) 835-8098
Fax: (510) 835-8099
Web site: http://www.youthlaw.org

National Food Service Management Institute
P.O. Drawer 188
University, MS 38677-0188
Tel: (601) 232-7658
Fax: (601) 232-5615
Web site: http://www.olemiss.edu/depts/nfsmi

National Healthy Mothers, Healthy Babies Coalition
121 North Washington Street, Suite 300
Alexandria, VA 22314
Tel: (703) 836-6110
Fax: (703) 836-3470
Web site: http://www.hmhb.org

National Maternal and Child Health Clearinghouse
2070 Chain Bridge Road, Suite 450
Vienna, VA 22182-2536
Tel: (703) 356-1964, (888) 434-4MCH
Fax: (703) 821-2098
Web site: http://www.nmchc.org

National Parent Teacher Association
330 North Wabash Avenue, Suite 2100
Chicago, IL 60611-3690
Tel: (312) 670-6782
Fax: (312) 670-6783
Web site: http://www.pta.org

National School Boards Association
1680 Duke Street
Alexandria, VA 22314
Tel: (703) 838-6722
Fax: (703) 683-7590
Web site: http://www.nsba.org

Society for Nutrition Education
7101 Wisconsin Avenue, Suite 901
Bethesda, MD 20814
Tel: (301) 656-4938
Fax: (301) 656-4958
Web site: http://www.sne.org

U.S. Department of Agriculture

Center for Nutrition Policy and Promotion
1120 20th Street, N.W., Suite 200 North
Washington, DC 20036-3406
Tel: (202) 418-2312
Fax: (202) 208-2321
Web site: http://www.usda.gov/cnpp

Cooperative State Research, Education, and Extension
  Service
1400 Independence Avenue, S.W.
South Building, Stop 2207, Room 3328
Washington, DC 20250-0900
Tel: (202) 720-4651
Fax: (202) 690-0289
Web site: http://www.reeusda.gov

Expanded Food and Nutrition Education Program
1400 Independence Avenue, S.W.
South Building, Stop 2225, Room 3444
Washington, DC 20250-2225
Tel: (202) 720-8067
Fax: (202) 690-2469
Web site: http://www.reeusda.gov/
4h/efnep/home.htm

Food and Nutrition Service
3101 Park Center Drive, Room 503
Alexandria, VA 22302-1500
Tel: (703) 305-2554
Fax: (703) 305-2576
Web site: http://www.fns.usda.gov/fns

Office of Analysis, Nutrition and Evaluation
Room 609
Tel: (703) 305-2554
Fax: (703) 305-2549

Special Supplemental Food Program Division
Room 540
Tel: (703) 305-2746
Fax: (703) 305-2196

National Agricultural Library
Food and Nutrition Information Center
10301 Baltimore Avenue, Room 304
Beltsville, MD 20705-2351
Tel: (301) 504-5719
Fax: (301) 504-6409
Web site: http://www.nal.usda.gov/fnic

U.S. Department of Health and Human Services

Centers for Disease Control and Prevention
1600 Clifton Road, N.E., E72
Atlanta, GA 30333
Tel: (800) 311-3435
Fax: (404) 639-6290
Web site: http://www.cdc.gov

Food and Drug Administration
Office of Consumer Affairs
5600 Fishers Lane, HFE-88, Room 16-85
Rockville, MD 20857
Tel: (301) 827-4422, (888) 463-6332
Fax: (301) 443-9767
Web site: http://www.fda.gov

Food and Drug Administration
Office of Food Labeling
200 C Street, S.W., Suite 1832
Washington, DC 20204
Tel: (202) 205-4561
Fax: (202) 205-4594
Web site: http://www.fda.gov

Health Resources and Services Administration
Maternal and Child Health Bureau
5600 Fishers Lane
Parklawn Building, Room 18-20
Rockville, MD 20857
Tel: (301) 443-0205
Fax: (301) 443-1797
Web site: http://www.mchb.hrsa.gov

Indian Health Service
Nutrition Services
5600 Fishers Lane
Parklawn Building, Room 6A-55
Rockville, MD 20857
Tel: (301) 443-1114
Fax: (301) 594-6213
Web site: http://www.ihs.gov

National Center for Health Statistics
Centers for Disease Control and Prevention
6525 Belcrest Road
Presidential Building, Room 1064
Hyattsville, MD 20782
Tel: (301) 436-8500
Web site: http://www.cdc.gov/nchs

National Institutes of Health
National Institute of Child Health
  and Human Development
31 Center Drive
Building 31, Room 2A-32, MSC 2425
Bethesda, MD 20892-2425
Tel: (301) 496-5133
Fax: (301) 496-7101
Web site: http://www.nichd.nih.gov

National Institutes of Health
National Institute of Diabetes and Digestive
  and Kidney Diseases
Division of Nutrition Research Coordination
9000 Rockville Pike
Building 45, Room 5AN-32, MSC 6600
Bethesda, MD 20892-6600
Tel: (301) 594-8822
Fax: (301) 480-3768
Web site: http://www.ep.niddk.nih.gov/
  divisions/dnrc/dnrchome.htm

Office of Disease Prevention and Health Promotion
200 Independence Avenue, S.W.
Hubert H. Humphrey Building, Room 738-G
Washington, DC 20201
Tel: (202) 205-8611
Fax: (202) 205-9478
Web site: http://www.odphp.osophs.dhhs.gov

Specific Nutrition Issues and Concerns

Breastfeeding

The Academy of Breastfeeding Medicine
P.O. Box 15945-284
Lenexa, KS 66285-5945
Tel: (913) 541-9077
Fax: (913) 541-0156
Web site: http://bfmed.org

Best Start
3500 East Fletcher Avenue, Suite 519
Tampa, FL 33613
Tel: (813) 971-2119, (800) 277-4975
Fax: (813) 971-2280

International Lactation Consultant Association
4101 Lake Boone Trail, Suite 201
Raleigh, NC 27607
Tel: (919) 787-5181
Fax: (919) 787-4916
Web site: http://www.ilca.org

La Leche League International
1400 North Meacham Road
Schaumburg, IL 60173-4048
Tel: (847) 519-7730, (800) 525-3243
Fax: (847) 519-0035
Web site: http://www.lalecheleague.org

Children and Adolescents with Special Health Care Needs

American Association of Mental Retardation
444 North Capitol Street, N.W., Suite 846
Washington, DC 20001-1512
Tel: (202) 387-1968, (800) 424-3688
Fax: (202) 387-2193
Web site: http://www.aamr.org

Easter Seals
230 West Monroe Street, Suite 1800
Chicago, IL 60606
Tel: (312) 726-6200, (800) 221-6827
Fax: (312) 726-1494
Web site: http://www.easter-seals.org

Family Voices
P.O. Box 769
Algodones, NM 87001
Tel: (505) 867-2368, (888) 835-5669
Fax: (505) 867-6517
Web site: http://www.familyvoices.org

March of Dimes
1275 Mamaroneck Avenue
White Plains, NY 10605
Tel: (914) 428-7100, (888) MODIMES
Fax: (914) 428-8203
Web site: http://www.modimes.org

National Information Center
   for Children and Youth with Disabilities
P.O. Box 1492
Washington, DC 20013-1492
Tel: (202) 884-8200, (800) 695-0285
Fax: (202) 884-8441
Web site: http://www.nichcy.org

National Parent Network on Disabilities
1130 17th Street, N.W., Suite 400
Washington, DC 20036
Tel: (202) 463-2299
Fax: (202) 463-9403
Web site: http://www.npnd.org

Diabetes Mellitus

American Diabetes Association
1701 North Beauregard Street
Alexandria, VA 22311
Tel: (703) 549-1500, (800) 342-2383
Fax: (703) 549-6995
Web site: http://www.diabetes.org

International Diabetes Center
3800 Park Nicollet Boulevard
Minneapolis, MN 55416
Tel: (612) 993-3393
Fax: (612) 993-1302
Web site: http://www.idcdiabetes.com

Juvenile Diabetes Foundation International
120 Wall Street, 19th Floor
New York, NY 10005-4001
Tel: (212) 785-9500, (800) 533-2873
Fax: (212) 785-9595
Web site: http://www.jdf.org/index.html

National Diabetes Information Clearinghouse
1 Information Way
Bethesda, MD 20892-3560
Tel: (301) 654-3327
Fax: (301) 907-8906
Web site: http://www.niddk.nih.gov/health/
   diabetes/ndic.htm

Eating Disorders

American Anorexia Bulimia Association
165 West 46th Street, Suite 1108
New York, NY 10036
Tel: (212) 575-6200
Fax: (212) 501-0342
Web site: http://www.aabainc.org/home.html

Anorexia Nervosa and Related Eating Disorders
P.O. Box 5102
Eugene, OR 97405
Tel: (541) 344-1144, (800) 931-2237
Web site: http://www.anred.com

National Association of Anorexia Nervosa
   and Associated Disorders
P.O. Box 7
Highland Park, IL 60035
Tel: (847) 831-3438
Fax: (847) 433-4632
Web site: http://www.anad.org

Food Allergies

American Academy of Allergy, Asthma
   and Immunology
611 East Wells Street
Milwaukee, WI 53202
Tel: (414) 272-6071, (800) 822-2762
Fax: (414) 272-6070
Web site: http://www.aaaai.org

Food Allergy Network
10400 Easton Place, Suite 107
Fairfax, VA 22030-2208
Tel: (703) 691-3179
Fax: (703) 691-2713
Web site: http://www.foodallergy.org

National Institute of Allergy and Infectious Diseases
9000 Rockville Pike
Building 31, Room 7A-50, MSC 2520
Bethesda, MD 20892-2520
Tel: (301) 496-5717
Fax: (301) 402-0120
Web site: http://www.niaid.nih.gov

Hyperlipidemia

American Heart Association
7272 Greenville Avenue
Dallas, TX 75231-4596
Tel: (214) 373-6300, (800) 242-8721
Fax: (214) 373-0268
Web site: http://www.americanheart.org

Hypertension

American Society of Hypertension
515 Madison Avenue, Suite 1212
New York, NY 10022
Tel: (212) 644-0650
Fax: (212) 644-0658
Web site: http://www.ash-us.org

Nutrition and Sports

American Alliance for Health, Physical Education, Recreation, and Dance
1900 Association Drive
Reston, VA 20191-1599
Tel: (703) 476-3400, (800) 213-7193
Fax: (703) 476-9572
Web site: http://www.aahperd.org

American College of Sports Medicine
401 West Michigan Street
Indianapolis, IN 46206-3233
Tel: (317) 637-9200
Fax: (317) 634-7817
Web site: http://www.acsm.org

Disabled Sports USA
451 Hungerford Drive, Suite 100
Rockville, MD 20850
Tel: (301) 217-0960
Fax: (301) 217-0968
Web site: www.dsusa.org

International Center for Sports Nutrition
502 South 44th Street, Suite 3012-NT
Omaha, NE 68105
Tel: (402) 559-5505
Fax: (402) 559-7302

National Association for Sport and Physical Education
1900 Association Drive
Reston, VA 20191-1598
Tel: (703) 476-3410, (800) 213-7193, ext. 410
Fax: (703) 476-8316
Web site: http://www.aahperd.org/naspe/naspe-main.html

National Association of Governor's Councils on Physical Fitness and Sports
201 South Capitol Avenue, Suite 560
Indianapolis, IN 46225
Tel: (317) 237-5630
Fax: (317) 237-5632
Web site: http://www.physicalfitness.org

National Recreation and Park Association
22377 Belmont Ridge Road
Ashburn, VA 20148
Tel: (703) 858-0784
Fax: (703) 858-0794
Web site: http://www.nrpa.org

National Sports Center for the Disabled
P.O. Box 1290
Winter Park, CO 80482
Tel: (970) 726-1540
Fax: (970) 726-4112
Web site: http://www.nscd.org

President's Council on Physical Fitness and Sports
200 Independence Avenue, S.W.
Hubert H. Humphrey Building, Room 738-H
Washington, DC 20201
Tel: (202) 690-9000
Fax: (202) 690-5211
Web site: http://www.indiana.edu/~preschal/
council.html

Special Olympics International
1325 G Street, N.W., Suite 500
Washington, DC 20005
Tel: (202) 628-3630
Fax: (202) 824-0200
Web site: http://www.specialolympics.org

Obesity

Shape Up America!
6707 Democracy Boulevard, Suite 306
Bethesda, MD 20817
Tel: (301) 493-5368
Fax: (301) 493-9504
Web site: http://www.shapeup.org

Weight-Control Information Network
1 WIN Way
Bethesda, MD 20892-3665
Tel: (301) 984-7378, (800) WIN-8098
Fax: (301) 984-7196
Web site: http://www.niddk.nih.gov/health/
nutrit/win.htm

Oral Health

American Academy of Pediatric Dentistry
211 East Chicago Avenue, Suite 700
Chicago, IL 60611-2663
Tel: (312) 337-2169
Fax: (312) 337-6329
Web site: http://www.aapd.org

American Dental Association
211 East Chicago Avenue
Chicago, IL 60611-2678
Tel: (312) 440-2500
Fax: (312) 440-2800
Web site: http://www.ada.org

American Dental Hygienists' Association
444 North Michigan Avenue, Suite 3400
Chicago, IL 60611
Tel: (312) 440-8900
Fax: (312) 440-6780
Web site: http://www.adha.org

Vegetarian Nutrition

The Vegetarian Resource Group
P.O. Box 1463
Baltimore, MD 21203
Tel: (410) 366-8343
Fax: (410) 366-8804
Web site: http://www.vrg.org

APPENDIX K

Appendix K: Federal Food Assistance and Nutrition Programs

Food Assistance and Nutrition Programs	Service Providers	Who Qualifies	Services/ Benefits	Funding	Administrative Agencies
National School Lunch Program (NSLP)					
Provides nutritious, low-cost lunches to children/adolescents enrolled in school	Participating public and nonprofit private schools	All children/adolescents attending school: Reduced-price lunches are available if family income is between 130% and 185% of the federal poverty level; free lunches are available if income is at or below 130% of the federal poverty level	Nutritious lunches at full or reduced prices, or free	USDA	State education agencies; local school districts
School Breakfast Program					
Provides nutritious, low-cost breakfasts to children/adolescents enrolled in school	Participating public and nonprofit private schools	All children/adolescents attending school: Reduced-price breakfasts are available if family income is between 130% and 185% of the federal poverty level; free breakfasts are available if income is at or below 130% of the federal poverty level	Nutritious breakfasts at full or reduced prices, or free	USDA	State education agencies; local school districts
Special Milk Program (SMP)					
Provides milk to children/adolescents enrolled in child care centers, summer camps, and schools that do not participate in other federal child nutrition meal-service programs	Child care centers, summer camps, and schools	All children/adolescents attending participating child care centers, summer camps, and schools	Milk at reduced prices, or free	USDA	State education agencies; local school districts

Food Assistance and Nutrition Programs	Service Providers	Who Qualifies	Services/ Benefits	Funding	Administrative Agencies
Summer Food Service Program (SFSP)					
Provides nutritious meals and snacks to children/adolescents in the summer, when the National School Lunch Program and School Breakfast Program are not operating	Public and nonprofit private schools; public and nonprofit private residential facilities; local, municipal, and county governments	Children/adolescents younger than 18 and people older than 18 who have disabilities and participate in county government–sponsored programs	Nutritious breakfasts, lunches, and/or snacks	USDA	State education agencies; local sponsors
Child and Adult Care Food Program (CACFP)					
Provides financial assistance to child and adult care centers so that they can provide nutritious meals to participants	Licensed child care centers, home-based child care centers, and adult care centers; Head Start programs; emergency shelters	Children 12 and younger; children/adolescents 15 and younger whose parents are migrant workers; people with physical/mental disabilities who receive care from centers in which the majority of participants are 18 or younger; adults with functional impairments	Free or reduced-price meals for children and adults in care centers; free meals for children in home-based child care centers; reimburse-ments to centers for providing up to two meals and one snack daily to each participant	USDA	State education agencies; local providers
Head Start					
Provides health, medical, dental, and nutrition services and educational, social, and other services to preschool children and their families if income is low	Local Head Start programs	Children 3–5 and their families receiving public assistance or with incomes below 100% of the federal poverty level; at least 10% of total enrollment available for children with disabilities	Health, medical, dental, and nutrition services and educational, social, and other services through assessment, early intervention, and prevention; nutritious meals and snacks (through the USDA Child and Adult Care Food Program); nutrition education; family counseling; referrals for social services	DHHS	DHHS regional offices; local providers

Food Assistance and Nutrition Programs	Service Providers	Who Qualifies	Services/ Benefits	Funding	Administrative Agencies
Early Head Start					
Provides health, medical, dental, and nutrition services and educational, social, and other services to women, children, and families	Local Early Head Start programs	Pregnant women with low incomes and children newborn to 3 years and their families receiving public assistance or with incomes below 100% of the federal poverty level; at least 10% of total enrollment available for children with disabilities	Health, medical, dental, and nutrition services and educational, social, and other services through assessment, early intervention, and prevention; nutritious meals and snacks (through the USDA Child and Adult Care Food Program); nutrition education; family counseling; referrals for social services	DHHS	DHHS regional offices; local providers
Special Supplemental Nutrition Program for Women, Infants and Children (WIC)					
Provides supplemental food, nutrition education, and access to health care to pregnant, postpartum, and breastfeeding women with low incomes; infants and children at nutritional risk from families with low incomes	Health, social services, and community agencies	Women who are pregnant or 6 months postpartum; women who are breast-feeding infants up to 1 year; infants and children up to age 5 certified to be at nutritional risk; families with incomes at or below 185% of the federal poverty level	Monthly food or coupons for food (e.g., milk, cheese, eggs, fruit juice, cereal, peanut butter, legumes, infant formula, infant cereal); nutrition education; health screening; refer-rals for social services	USDA	State health agencies; local agencies
Commodity Supplemental Food Program (CSFP)					
Provides commodity foods to women, infants, children, and elderly people	Public and private nonprofit agencies (community health and social service agencies)	Pregnant, postpartum, or breastfeeding women and infants and children up to age 6 with incomes at or below 185% of the federal poverty level; elderly people at least 60 years of age with low incomes are eligible if their benefits do not reduce benefits to eligible women, infants, and children	Monthly commodity canned or packaged foods (e.g., fruit, vegetables, meat, infant formula, farina, beans, other foods as available)	USDA	State health agencies

Food Assistance and Nutrition Programs	Service Providers	Who Qualifies	Services/ Benefits	Funding	Administrative Agencies
Food Stamp Program (FSP)					
Provides assistance to people with low incomes to increase their ability to buy food	Local public assistance and social service agencies	U.S. citizens, refugees with visa status, legal aliens, and low-income households with resources (aside from income) of $2,000 or less ($3,000 or less if household has at least one person age 60 or older)	Coupons and benefits issued electronically for the purchase of foods at participating stores	USDA	State welfare, social service, and human service agencies
The Emergency Food Assistance Program (TEFAP)					
Provides commodity foods to households with low incomes	Public and private nonprofit agencies (community action agencies, councils on aging, local health and school districts)	Varies by state	Periodic distribution of food (e.g., canned and dried fruit, fruit juice, canned vegetables, meat, poultry, fish, rice, grits, cereal, peanut butter, nonfat dry milk, dried egg mix, pasta products)	USDA	State and local agencies
Nutrition Assistance Program (NAP) for Puerto Rico					
Provides money to participants for buying food and money for administrative costs, up to an amount established by the legislature	Puerto Rico	People living in Puerto Rico; eligibility rules similar to the Food Stamp Program	Cash to be used for food only	USDA	Puerto Rico
Food Distribution Programs on Indian Reservations (FDPIR)					
Provides commodity foods to families with low incomes as a substitute for the Food Stamp Program	Local agencies	Families with low incomes living on Indian reservations and Native American families residing in designated areas near reservations	Monthly commodity foods	USDA	Indian tribal councils

Food Assistance and Nutrition Programs	Service Providers	Who Qualifies	Services/ Benefits	Funding	Administrative Agencies
Elderly Nutrition Program (ENP)					
Provides meals and nutrition education to the elderly	Area agencies on aging; other providers of services to people who are elderly	People 60 or older; people younger than 60 with disabilities who reside in housing occupied primarily by people who are elderly; spouses of eligible people	Nutritious meals; nutrition education; access to social and rehabilitative services; transportation	DHHS; states; individual donations	State and local agencies on aging
Expanded Food and Nutrition Education Program (EFNEP)					
Provides nutrition education to people with low incomes	Local Cooperative Extension Service offices where program is available	Families with incomes at or below 125% of the federal poverty level and with children/adolescents younger than 19 who are at risk for inadequate nutrition	Education and training on food and nutrition for families	USDA	State land grant universities; Cooperative Extension Service offices

Source: Adapted, with permission, from Table 4-3 of Kaufman M. 1990. *Nutrition in Public Health: A Handbook for Developing Programs and Services.* Gaithersburg, MD: Aspen Publishers. Copyright © 1990 Aspen Publishers, Inc.